BMA

MRCOG: Part 2 MCQs

Clinical Obstetrics and Gynaecology

Edited by
Khaldoun W Sharif and Joseph A Jordan

MRCOG: Part 2 MCQs

Clinical Obstetrics and Gynaecology

Edited by

Khaldoun W Sharif MRCOG, MFFP, FICS,

Lecturer, Medical School, University of Birmingham;
Senior Registrar in Obstetrics and Gynaecology,
Birmingham Women's Hospital, Edgbaston
Birmingham, UK.

Joseph A Jordan MD, FRCOG,

Consultant Gynaecologist, and Medical Director
Birmingham Women's Hospital, Edgbaston
Birmingham, UK.

W.B. Saunders Company Ltd

London • Philadelphia • Toronto • Sydney • Tokyo

W.B. Saunders Company Ltd 24–28 Oval Road,
London NW1 7DX, UK

The Curtis Center
Independence Square West
Philadelphia, PA 19106–3399, USA

Harcourt Brace & Company
55 Horner Avenue
Toronto, Ontario M8Z 4X6, Canada

Harcourt Brace & Company, Australia
30–52 Smidmore Street
Marrickville, NSW 2204, Australia

Harcourt Brace, Japan
Ichibancho Central Building,
22–1 Ichibancho
Chiyoda-ku, Tokyo, 102, Japan

A catalogue record for this book is available from the British Library

ISBN 0–7020–2120–2

Typeset by Laserscript, Mitcham, Surrey
Printed in Great Britain by
WBC Book Manufacturing, Bridgend, Mid Glamorgan

Contents

Contributors

Abukhalil, I.H. MRCOG, Lecturer in Obstetrics and Gynaecology, Birmingham Women's Hospital, Birmingham.

Adeghe, J. PhD, MRCOG, Consultant Obstetrician and Gynaecologist, New Cross Hospital, Wolverhampton.

Afnan, M.A. MRCOG, Senior Lecturer in Obstetrics and Gynaecology, Birmingham Women's Hospital, Birmingham.

Ashok, P. MRCOG, Sp. Registrar in Obstetrics and Gynaecology, City Hospital, Birmingham.

Beattie, R.B. MD, MRCOG, Consultant in Fetal Medicine, University Hospital of Wales, Cardiff.

Bilalis, D. MRCOG, Research Fellow in Assisted Conception, Birmingham Women's Hospital, Birmingham.

Blunt, S. MD, MRCOG, Consultant Obstetrician and Gynaecologist, Birmingham Women's Hospital, Birmingham.

Burckhill, L. MRCPsych, MFFP, Director, Brook Advisory Centre, Birmingham.

Chan, K.K. FRCOG, FRCS, Consultant Gynaecologist, Birmingham Women's Hospital, Birmingham.

Condie, R. MD, FRCOG, Consultant Obstetrician and Gynaecologist, City Hospital, Birmingham.

Cooper, G. FRCA, Senior Lecturer in Anaesthesia, Birmingham Women's Hospital, Birmingham.

Ebbiary, N.A. MD, MRCOG, Consultant Obstetrician and Gynaecologist, Blackburn General Hospital, Blackburn.

El-Mardi, A.A. MRCOG, MFFP, FICS, MMed (O&G), Staff Grade Obstetrician and Gynaecologist, Good Hope Hospital, Sutton Coldfield.

Emens, J.M. MD, FRCOG, Consultant Gynaecologist, Birmingham Women's Hospital, Birmingham.

Farndon, P. BSc, MD, FRCP, DCH, Professor of Clinical Genetics, Birmingham Women's Hospital, Birmingham.

Gee, H. MD, FRCOG, Consultant Obstetricia/Director of Postgraduate Training, Birmingham Women's Hospital, Birmingham.

Harrison, G. FRCA, Consultant Anaesthetist, Birmingham Women's Hospital, Birmingham.

Jordan, J.A. MD, FRCOG, Consultant Gynaecologist and Medical Director, Birmingham Women's Hospital, Birmingham.

Kelly, J. FRCOG, FRCS, Senior Lecturer in Obstetrics and Gynaecology, Birmingham Women's Hospital, Birmingham.

Khalaf. Y. MSc, MD, MRCOG, Lecturer in Obstetrics and Gynaecology, St Thomas's Hospital, London.

Kilby, M. MD, MRCOG, Senior Lecturer in Fetal Medicine, Birmingham Women's Hospital, Birmingham.

Lashen, H. MRCOG, Research Fellow in Assisted Conception, Birmingham Women's Hospital, Birmingham.

Lewis, M. FRCA, Consultant Anaesthetist, Birmingham Women's Hospital, Birmingham.

Luesley, D.M. MD, FRCOG, Professor of Gynaecological Oncology, City Hospital, Birmingham.

Mann, M. MRCOG, Senior Registrar in Community Gynaecology, Birmingham Women's Hospital, Birmingham.

McHugo, J. FRCP, FRCR, Consultant Radiologist, Birmingham Women's Hospital, Birmingham.

Morgan, I. FRCP, Consultant Neonatologist, Birmingham Women's Hospital, Birmingham.

Murphy, C. MRCOG, FRCS, Consultant Obstetrician and Gynaecologist, City Hospital, Birmingham.

Newton, J.R. MD, LLM, MFFP, FRCOG, Professor and Head, Academic Department of Obstetrics and Gynaecology, Birmingham Women's Hospital, Birmingham.

Nicholson, H.O. FRCOG, FRCS, Consultant Obstetrician and Gynaecologist, Birmingham Women's Hospital, Birmingham.

Penketh, R. BSc, MD, MRCOG, Consultant Obstetrician and Gynaecologist, University Hospital of Wales, Cardiff.

Persad, P. MRCOG, MRCPI, DFFP, Research Fellow in Obstetrics and Gynaecology, Solihull Hospital, Solihull.

Pogmore, J.R. FRCOG, Consultant Obstetrician and Gynaecologist, Birmingham Women's Hospital, Birmingham.

Rollason, T. FRCPath, Consultant Pathologist, Birmingham Women's Hospital, Birmingham.

Sawers, R.S. FRCOG, Consultant Obstetrician and Gynaecologist, Birmingham Women's Hospital, Birmingham.

Sharif, K.W. MRCOG, MFFP, FICS, Lecturer in Obstetrics and Gynaecology, Birmingham Women's Hospital, Birmingham.

Stewart, P. MD, FRCP, Professor of Medicine, Queen Elizabeth Medical Centre, Birmingham.

Weaver, J.B. MD, FRCOG, FRCS, Consultant Obstetrician, Birmingham Women's Hospital, Birmingham.

Whittle, M.J. MD, FRCOG, FRCP, Professor of Fetal Medicine, Birmingham Women's Hospital, Birmingham.

Williams, D. FIBMS, Manager of Cytology Laboratories, Birmingham Women's Hospital, Birmingham.

Wood, L. MRCOG, FRCS, Consultant Obstetrician and Gynaecologist, Walsgrave Hospital, Coventry.

Preface

Multiple choice questions (MCQs) are here to stay! They form part of most undergraduate and postgraduate medical examinations in the UK, because they allow testing of a wide base of knowledge over a relatively short period of time and lend themselves easily to objective and quick marking. MCQs form part of the Part 2 examination of the Membership of the Royal College of Obstetricians and Gynaecologists (MRCOG), and this book is written primarily for candidates preparing for this exam.

The MRCOG Part 2 MCQ paper consists of 300 questions. This book contains 400 one-stem/5-branch MCQs, thus providing 2000 separate questions, together with their correct answers and explanatory notes. The MCQs have been divided into the recognized main four subspecialties: Perinatal Medicine, Reproductive Medicine, Gynaecological Oncology, and Medical and Surgical Gynaecology. The questions themselves provide a means of testing knowledge and revision, whereas the explanatory notes will aid learning and the retention of facts. Most questions are pitched at MRCOG level. Although some might appear too easy and others rather difficult, this is actually how the questions appear in the real exam. After all, the usual definition of an easy question is one to which the candidate knows the correct answer – a rather 'loose' subjective definition. The aim of this book is to make more exam questions easy for you!

Our task in editing this book has been made much easier and more enjoyable by the invaluable help of our contributors. They are active clinicians at the forefront of busy clinical practice and research, and many are senior MRCOG examiners. They span the different specialties of Anaesthesia, Surgery, Medicine, Neonatology, Pathology, Genetics, Radiology, as well as Obstetrics and Gynaecology and their different subspecialties. All of them have worked at the

Birmingham Women's Hospital and thus provide a coherent and balanced view of the different clinical problems based on experience at one of the busiest tertiary referral centres in the UK.

K.W.S.
J.A.J.

1

How to Answer Multiple Choice Questions in Part 2 of the MRCOG Examination

The Multiple Choice Question (MCQ) paper of Part 2 of the Membership Examination consists of 300 true-or-false MCQs in book form. The time allowed is two hours. Each item correctly answered (i.e. a true statement indicated as true or a false statement indicated as false) is awarded one mark (+1). For each incorrect answer no mark (0) is awarded. All items must be answered true or false. Incorrect answers are not penalized; there is no negative marking. The questions are in the form of stems, each followed by a *variable* number of branches, and the stem taken together with each branch is counted as a single question. This is different from the usual MCQ style where every stem is always followed by five branches. However, the one-stem/five-branch style is used in this book as it allows more questions to be asked about each subject, and hence more practice.

The following specimen questions and answers illustrate what you will find in the Part 2 MCQ paper:

Cholestasis of pregnancy is associated with:

1 preterm labour
2 increased perinatal mortality
3 increased incidence of postpartum haemorrhage

Transverse lie of the second twin at term:

4 is an absolute indication for caesarean section

Uterine curettage:

5 is associated with an increased incidence of placenta praevia in a subsequent pregnancy
6 is important in the investigation of secondary infertility

At the end of this book (in the appendix) you will find a copy of the Detailed Instructions and Sample Answer Sheet for the MCQ Papers in the Part 2 MRCOG Examination.

MCQ Techniques

The following guidelines should assist you in answering the questions correctly.

Read Carefully and Understand Clearly

Read the question carefully and make sure you understand it. Do not simply *think* you understand it. In the Part 2 MRCOG, when you have to go through 300 items in two hours, it is not uncommon to rush in and misread the questions. 'Pre-eclampsia' could be easily misread as 'eclampsia', 'morbidity' as 'mortality', and 'fetal haemoglobin' as 'fetal blood'. The opening stem should be read together with each of the branches and taken as a single item. Each item should be considered independently of the other statements.

Do Not Read Between the Lines

Accept the question at face value and do not look for catches or hidden meanings. Trust that the examiners are trying to test your factual knowledge, not to trick you into making mistakes. What you clearly understand from the question is what is meant by it.

To Guess or Not To Guess

After reading (and understanding) each item, your initial response will fall into one of three categories.

First, you may be sure of the answer and have no doubt about the correct response (whether true or false) – go ahead and without hesitation answer the question.

Second, there are items about which you are not quite certain and yet they 'ring a bell'. You may not know the answer immediately, but from your basic knowledge you could reason it out from first principles – go for it and play your hunches. Such educated hunches that are based on sound judgement and reasoning are more often right than wrong, and you are advised to be bold and answer these items accordingly.

Third, you may be totally ignorant of the answer. The usual advice in such situations, with the *negative* marking system used in many MCQ examinations, is not to guess. However, in the Part 2 MRCOG examination this system has been abolished since 1994. There is nothing to be lost by blindly guessing the answers to such items. If you are incorrect you will not lose any marks and if you are correct (50% probability) you will gain. Readers who are preparing for other examinations that still use the negative marking system should not guess blindly.

Organize Your Time

In the Part 2 MRCOG Examination you are allowed two hours for 300 questions. This might appear too little, but it is not. The items you are sure of will take only a few seconds. The same applies to items about which you are totally ignorant. We suggest you go through the whole paper first, answering questions to which you are sure you know the answers. As you are unlikely to change these answers, you are advised to record them on the answer sheet from the outset. The remaining time should be directed to the unanswered, more time-consuming, items about which you are uncertain but have enough basic knowledge to make reasoned hunches. You should have marked these items on the question paper during your first reading to facilitate coming back to them. Any remaining time should be spent on revising the answers, but remember that your first thought is likely to be the correct answer.

Fill in the Answer Sheet Correctly

A sure recipe for disaster in MCQ examinations is to make a systematic error in recording the answers. If you answer question 1 in place of question 2, all the following answers will also be recorded wrongly. Such mistakes are quite easily done under the stress of the examination. Make sure when you fill in every answer that it is in the right place.

MCQ Terminology

Candidates may find difficulty in understanding some words commonly used in MCQs. The following is a guide to the accepted meanings of some of these troublesome words:

- Common/characteristic/usual/typical: what is expected to be found in the average textbook description.
- Recognized/may occur/can occur: has been described, even if rarely.
- Essential feature: must occur to make a diagnosis.
- Frequently/often: imply a rate of occurrence greater than 50%.
- Never: 0%.
- Always: 100%.
- Rare: <5%.

Beware that absolutes are very rare in medicine. Items that contain always or never are often false.

2

Perinatal Medicine

Questions

1. **Regarding 'HELLP' syndrome:**
   A. in its original description the 'H' stood for haemolysis.
   B. it cannot be diagnosed if the platelet count is $>100{,}000/\text{mm}^3$.
   C. alkaline phosphatase levels are always markedly raised.
   D. eclampsia has been reported in about 15% of cases.
   E. the recurrence rate in a subsequent pregnancy is usually less than 5%.

2. **Maternal cardiac output during pregnancy:**
   A. alters little until about 18 weeks of pregnancy.
   B. will increase to about 40–50% of its pre-pregnancy value by about term.
   C. can be enhanced by the use of epidural anaesthesia.
   D. will, in the presence of mitral stenosis, fall in the second stage of labour.
   E. returns immediately to pre-pregnancy levels following delivery of the placenta.

3. **Routine antenatal ultrasonography performed at or before 20 weeks:**
   A. will effectively replace maternal serum α-fetoprotein (AFP) in the assessment of the fetal neural tube.
   B. will help to identify close to 90% of serious cardiac anomalies.
   C. is unreliable in predicting placental site.
   D. is a good time to assess chorionicity in twins.
   E. indicates a 50% risk of Down's syndrome if isolated choroid plexus cysts are detected.

4. Maternal nephrotic syndrome is associated with:
- **A.** renal vein thrombosis.
- **B.** urolithiasis.
- **C.** adult polycystic renal disease.
- **D.** essential hypertension.
- **E.** antiphospholipid syndrome.

5. The fetal biophysical profile (BPP) may have useful reliable applications in the following clinical circumstances:
- **A.** insulin-dependent diabetes mellitus.
- **B.** a pregnancy at 42 weeks.
- **C.** multiple pregnancy.
- **D.** maternal hypertensive disorder.
- **E.** preterm rupture of the membranes.

6. The following statements are true about insulin-dependent diabetes and pregnancy:
- **A.** Unexplained intrauterine death remains a leading cause of perinatal mortality.
- **B.** The deterioration in diabetic nephropathy that occurs in pregnancy persists postpartum.
- **C.** Caesarean section rate is usually about 30–50% in most series.
- **D.** The risk of intrauterine growth restriction (IUGR) correlates to the glycosylated haemoglobin (HbA_1C) level.
- **E.** The commonest structural abnormality in offspring of diabetics is caudal regression syndrome.

7. The following statements are true about Rhesus (Rh) disease:
- **A.** Anti-D given in adequate amounts following delivery is effective in all but about 5% of cases.
- **B.** A maternal anti-D level of less than 10 iu/ml does not indicate the need for further investigation.
- **C.** Amniotic fluid spectroscopic characteristics are determined at a wavelength of 400 A.
- **D.** Amniotic fluid polymerase chain reaction (PCR) can now be used to establish fetal Rh type.
- **E.** Maternal anti-D prophylaxis at 28 and 34 weeks does appear effective in reducing sensitization.

8. The following ultrasonographic measurements provide reliable pregnancy dating information (± 7 days):

A. crown-rump length at 9 weeks.
B. femur length at 28 weeks.
C. head/trunk ratio at 18 weeks.
D. cerebellar diameter at 22 weeks.
E. gestation sac diameter at 13 weeks.

9. The antihypertensive drug:

A. hydralazine blocks calcium channels.
B. methyldopa can cause depression.
C. atenolol, when used in essential hypertension, has been associated with IUGR.
D. captopril is safe in pregnancy.
E. nifedipine can be used sublingually for rapid control of hypertension.

10. The following statements are true about fetal isoimmune erythroblastic anaemia:

A. Anti-Kell disease cannot be monitored reliably by amniocentesis.
B. A pregnancy with a different partner makes past obstetric history unreliable.
C. Anti-D is significant only above 15 iu/ml.
D. Doppler waveforms in the umbilical artery may predict anaemia.
E. In the 'mirror syndrome' the mother develops pre-eclampsia.

11. A 20-week anomaly scan will detect the following percentage of anomalies:

A. over 80% of open spina bifidas.
B. 60% of trisomies.
C. 30% of cardiac anomalies.
D. 90% of cases of duodenal atresia.
E. 80% of cleft lips.

12. With the use of low-dose aspirin in pregnancy:

A. platelet thromboxane synthesis in the presystemic circulation is inhibited.

B. large multicentre trials indicate the benefit of low-dose aspirin prophylaxis for all patients who had pre-eclampsia in a previous pregnancy.

C. clinical trials have shown that aspirin has no effect on the incidence of venous thromboembolism in pregnancy.

D. to be most effective, low-dose aspirin (as prophylaxis) for pre-eclampsia has to be started before 16 weeks' gestation.

E. epidural anaesthesia is contraindicated when low-dose aspirin has been given.

13. Regarding metabolism in the small for gestational age fetus:

A. these fetuses exhibit hypertriglyceridaemia.

B. plasma insulin levels are increased.

C. the glycine to valine ratio is increased.

D. plasma cortisol levels are increased.

E. plasma glucose concentrations are increased.

14. The following is true of the coagulation and the fibrinolytic system in pregnancy:

A. Platelets release thromboxane A_2.

B. Plasma fibrinogen concentrations decrease with gestation.

C. There is a rise in Factor VIII antigen:activity ratio.

D. Angiotensin II activates platelet function.

E. Arachidonic acid-induced platelet aggregation is reduced.

15. The vacuum extractor in assisted vaginal delivery:

A. should be used when the operator is not absolutely sure of the position of the fetal vertex in the second stage of labour.

B. is associated with significantly more maternal trauma than forceps delivery.

C. is associated with retinal haemorrhages in the fetus.

D. is more likely to be associated with a failed vaginal delivery than when forceps are applied.

E. can be utilized when the fetal head is two-fifths palpable abdominally in a multiparous patient.

16. Placental abruption:

A. is associated with preterm prelabour rupture of the membranes.
B. is associated with pre-eclampsia.
C. occurs in 1 of every 500 pregnancies.
D. is associated with crack cocaine consumption.
E. is associated with a recurrence rate of at least 10%.

17. The following statements concerning autoimmune thrombocytopenic purpura (ATP) are correct:

A. It is the most common autoimmune cause of bleeding in pregnancy.
B. It is characterized by the production of immunoglobulin (Ig) M antibodies directed against maternal and fetal platelets.
C. The spleen is the major site of antibody production.
D. Corticosteroids are the mainstay therapy in pregnant women.
E. High-dose immunoglobulin given intravenously has no effect on platelet counts.

18. Wound infection after caesarean section:

A. occurs overall in 5% of patients.
B. is associated with prolonged prelabour ruptured membranes.
C. is more common after a failed trial of forceps delivery.
D. is more likely to be prevented by peritoneal lavage with antibiotics than by systemic antibiotics.
E. in the form of necrotizing fasciitis commonly occurs within the first 48 hours of operation.

19. With regard to cytomegalovirus (CMV) infection in pregnancy:

A. it is an infection by a DNA virus.
B. the maternal infection is often 'silent'.
C. prognosis is poor for babies who have clinically apparent disease at birth.
D. the optimal indicator of intrauterine infection is anti-CMV IgA in fetal blood.
E. effective antiviral therapy exists for treatment.

20. In the fetus with a sacral coccygeal teratoma:
- **A.** there is a recognized association with polyhydramnios.
- **B.** diagnosis after 30 weeks' gestation is a poor prognostic sign.
- **C.** dystocia during labour is a recognized complication.
- **D.** malignant change is common.
- **E.** there is a recognized association with hydrops.

21. Diamniotic-monochorionic twins:
- **A.** have two separate placental masses.
- **B.** have more placental vascular anastomoses than in dichorionic placentation.
- **C.** may be complicated by twin–twin transfusion syndrome.
- **D.** comprise 70% of all monozygotic twins.
- **E.** have a perinatal mortality rate of approximately 25%.

22. With regard to human immunodeficiency virus (HIV):
- **A.** women comprise 11% of the total infected.
- **B.** 80% of cases of paediatric acquired immune deficiency syndrome (AIDS) are secondary to vertical transmission of HIV from mother to fetus.
- **C.** it is a DNA virus.
- **D.** seropositive women are more at risk of spontaneous miscarriage.
- **E.** the risk of transmission of infection transplacentally approaches 90%.

23. In rhesus disease of the newborn:
- **A.** anti-D antibodies are still the most common causative antibodies.
- **B.** red cell destruction by anti-D is complement mediated.
- **C.** the majority of affected babies require intrauterine intravascular transfusion.
- **D.** prevention may be by antenatal administration of rhesus immune globulin.
- **E.** high-dose immunoglobulin administration to severely alloimmunized pregnant women has improved perinatal survival.

24. Fetal 'programming' of human adult disease indicates that:

A. a small for dates baby has an increased risk of cardiovascular disease in adulthood.

B. birthweight predicts adult death rates more strongly than does weight at 1 year.

C. abdominal circumference at birth is inversely related to serum cholesterol concentration in adulthood.

D. placental type 2, 11β-hydroxysteroid dehydrogenase activity is directly correlated with placental weight.

E. placental weight is positively correlated with death from cardiovascular disease in adulthood.

25. In the ultrasonographic detection of intrauterine growth restriction (IUGR):

A. umbilical artery Doppler waveforms are superior to abdominal circumference in the prediction of small for gestational age babies.

B. abdominal circumference alone is a good predictor of a small for gestational age neonate.

C. head circumference:abdominal circumference ratios are better predictors of small for gestational age neonates than abdominal circumference alone.

D. the middle cerebral artery Doppler pulsatility index has a greater prediction for small for gestational age babies at birth than umbilical artery pulsatility index.

E. ponderal index at birth is superior to birthweight in predicting neonatal complications associated with IUGR.

26. The following statements regarding hypertension in pregnancy are correct:

A. Rapid weight gain with oedema is diagnostic of pre-eclampsia.

B. A raised serum level of uric acid is predictive of pre-eclampsia.

C. Chronic hypertension is present in approximately 10% of pregnancies.

D. The rationale for the use of antihypertensive therapy in mild pre-eclampsia is to improve blood pressure.

E. Comparative trials between hydralazine, nifedipine and labetalol have not shown one agent to be superior in the acute management of severe hypertension in pregnancy.

27. The following statements regarding hypertensive disorders of pregnancy are correct:

A. The CLASP trial concluded that the use of prophylactic low-dose aspirin had no statistically significant effect on stillbirths or neonatal deaths.

B. CLASP concluded that low-dose aspirin might be of benefit in women judged to be especially liable to early-onset pre-eclampsia.

C. The incidence of HELLP syndrome in women with pre-eclampsia has been reported to vary between 15 and 25%.

D. The reported perinatal mortality rate associated with HELLP syndrome ranges from 2 to 6%.

E. Women with hypertensive disorders during pregnancy do not run an increased risk of chronic hypertension in later life.

28. The following are true concerning amniocentesis in the management of fetal isoimmune erythroblastosis:

A. It is of no value before 27 weeks' gestation.

B. It can be used to manage pregnancies complicated by anti-Kell antibodies.

C. When the amniotic fluid delta optical density (OD) is falling and the maternal antibodies are stable, the fetus is definitely rhesus negative and no further checks are necessary.

D. It is indicated when maternal anti-D concentration exceeds 4 iu/ml.

E. Rising delta OD indicates the need for immediate delivery.

29. Reliable information about the severity of rhesus disease could be obtained by:

A. ultrasonographic evidence of fetal subdiaphragmatic fluid.

B. a single amniotic fluid analysis for delta OD level.

C. past obstetric history involving a different partner.

D. a cordocentesis for fetal haemoglobin.

E. a maternal antibody level of 10 iu/ml.

30. Preterm labour has been associated with infection of the genital tract by:
A. *Neisseria gonorrhoea.*
B. *Chlamydia trachomatis.*
C. *Ureaplasma urealyticum.*
D. *Bacteroides.*
E. *Gardnerella vaginalis.*

31. In normal pregnancy the vagina shows:
A. an increase in the concentration of *Gardnerella vaginalis.*
B. an increased concentration of lactobacilli.
C. a decreased concentration of anaerobes.
D. a rise in pH.
E. a more homogeneous flora.

32. Induction of labour beyond 41 weeks' completed gestation:
A. increases the rate of instrumental deliveries.
B. increases caesarean section rates.
C. reduces perinatal mortality rate.
D. reduces meconium aspiration syndrome.
E. reduces the incidence of neonatal seizures.

33. Forceps delivery is:
A. associated with occult damage to the anal sphincter in up to four out of five cases.
B. associated with bowel symptoms in a third of cases.
C. recommended prophylactically for the cephalically presenting premature fetus.
D. associated with cephalhaematoma in the neonate.
E. associated with maternal facial palsy.

34. Amniotomy in labour:
A. speeds up progress.
B. reduces the need for caesarean section.
C. decreases analgesia requirements.
D. avoids the need for oxytocin.
E. improves neonatal outcome.

35. Reduction in the need for medical intervention in low-risk labour can be brought about by:

A. routine early amniotomy.
B. oxytocin infusion.
C. epidural analgesia.
D. continuous electronic fetal monitoring.
E. psychological support for the mother.

36. Amnio-infusion for oligohydramnios in labour:

A. reduces perinatal mortality rate.
B. reduces the incidence of variable decelerations.
C. reduces caesarean section rates.
D. increases the incidence of puerperal pyrexia.
E. reduces the risk of meconium aspiration.

37. External cephalic version performed at 37 weeks:

A. does not reduce surgical intervention rates.
B. does not affect the incidence of breech delivery.
C. carries a risk of uterine rupture.
D. is successful in over half the attempts.
E. should not be attempted in rhesus-negative women.

38. In a pregnant woman whose first and only delivery was by lower segment caesarean section for a breech presentation:

A. the chances of a vaginal delivery are over 60%.
B. the risk of scar rupture or dehiscence is over 1%.
C. erect lateral pelvimetry should be performed to exclude cephalopelvic disproportion.
D. intrauterine pressure monitoring has been shown to reduce the risk of uterine rupture.
E. continuous electronic fetal heart rate monitoring should be used in labour.

39. Signs suggestive of scar rupture or dehiscence in a patient who has had a previous lower segment caesarean section include:

A. vaginal bleeding.
B. poor progress.
C. haematuria.
D. maternal tachycardia.
E. abnormal CTG.

40. At about 6 weeks postnatally:
- **A.** women should have a routine vaginal examination.
- **B.** a cervical smear should be collected.
- **C.** over 50% of women would have resumed sexual intercourse.
- **D.** most women complaining of backache following delivery would have become asymptomatic.
- **E.** is the ideal time for starting the oral contraceptive pill.

41. There is a recognized association between breech presentation at term and:
- **A.** cornual implantation of the placenta.
- **B.** increased risk of fetal anomaly.
- **C.** placenta praevia.
- **D.** increased perinatal morbidity.
- **E.** previous history of breech presentation.

42. Clinical examination of the normal maternal heart in later pregnancy is likely to show:
- **A.** the apex beat in the 4th intercostal space.
- **B.** a systolic ejection murmur along the left border of the sternum.
- **C.** splitting of the first heart sound.
- **D.** occasional bouts of atrial fibrillation.
- **E.** ectopic beats.

43. Increased risk of thromboembolism in normal pregnancy is partly due to:
- **A.** reduced levels of antithrombin III.
- **B.** increased progesterone levels.
- **C.** raised levels of liver-produced clotting factors.
- **D.** reduced levels of protein S.
- **E.** changes in blood viscosity.

44. In normal pregnancy the increased renal glomerular filtration rate:
- **A.** can lead to renal glycosuria.
- **B.** decreases maternal serum urea and creatinine concentrations.
- **C.** starts in the second trimester.
- **D.** is in the order of 20–30%.
- **E.** predisposes to urinary tract infection.

45. In normal pregnancy:

A. the oxygen-carrying capacity of the blood rises by 15–20%.
B. the arteriovenous oxygen difference falls.
C. cardiac output rises by 30–40%.
D. a fall in haemoglobin concentration reflects anaemia.
E. dyspnoea on mild exertion is a common symptom in the third trimester.

46. Uterine inversion:

A. is associated with postpartum haemorrhage.
B. always occurs during delivery of the placenta.
C. requires urinary catheterization before attempting repositioning.
D. requires manual exploration of the uterus after repositioning.
E. has a recurrence rate of up to 50% in subsequent deliveries.

47. Amniotic fluid embolism:

A. is 8–10 times more common in women over 40 years old than in those in their 20s.
B. can occur only after the membranes have ruptured.
C. is diagnosed by the presence of fetal squames in the pulmonary capillary bed.
D. is associated with the use of oxytocin.
E. is more common in primigravidae.

48. After caesarean section for failure to progress in labour:

A. clinical pelvimetry should be performed.
B. radiographic pelvimetry (erect lateral) should be performed.
C. a review of the cervimetric pattern will give the exact cause.
D. the risk of postpartum depression is increased compared with that following spontaneous vaginal delivery.
E. the next delivery is best managed by elective caesarean section.

49. Bacteriuria in pregnancy:

A. is associated with lower socioeconomic status.
B. affects 15% of women.
C. if left untreated, will progress to symptomatic infection in about 75% of women.
D. should be treated with tetracycline.
E. is associated with increased risk of anaemia.

50. Dexon (polyglycolic acid) suture material:

A. is a co-polymer of lactide and glycotide.
B. is completely absorbed within 90–120 days.
C. evokes less tissue reaction than catgut.
D. has less tensile strength than Vicryl (polyglactin 910).
E. when used to suture episiotomy, produces significantly more pain than when catgut is used.

51. The obstetric forceps:

A. should not be used to assist delivery unless the fetus is presenting cephalically.
B. may be used in face presentation when the chin is directed towards the sacrum (mentoposterior).
C. can be used to assist delivery of the fetal head during caesarean section.
D. should be used routinely to assist vaginal delivery of the preterm infant.
E. should not be used unless the fetal head is engaged.

52. The vacuum extractor:

A. should be used for instrumental delivery if the fetal head position cannot be identified.
B. is available with a cup of one size only.
C. used with the Silastic cup for occipitoposterior position is associated with a higher failure rate compared with the rigid metal cup.
D. should be used with a vacuum of about 0.8 kg/cm^2.
E. is associated with more maternal trauma than the obstetric forceps.

53. Instrumental vaginal delivery:

A. is commoner in labouring women with epidural anaesthesia.
B. with the vacuum extractor is too slow to be useful when rapid delivery is required
C. with the vacuum extractor is significantly more likely to cause cephalhaematoma than the forceps.
D. may be avoided by the appropriate use of Syntocinon in the second stage of labour.
E. leads to third-degree perineal tears more frequently with forceps than with the vacuum extractor.

54. In caesarean sections:

A. the associated maternal mortality rate is about 3–4 per 10,000 procedures in the UK.

B. there is no relationship between abdominal incision size and difficulty of fetal delivery.

C. manual removal of the placenta increases maternal blood loss.

D. two-layer closure of the uterus leads to less blood loss and a stronger scar than one-layer closure.

E. suturing the uterus after bringing it out through the abdominal incision (exteriorization) leads to more blood loss than suturing it while within the pelvis.

55. Caesarean section:

A. in the UK is most commonly performed for dystocia (prolonged labour).

B. is safer than vaginal delivery for the preterm breech.

C. associated infection is markedly reduced by the use of prophylactic antibiotics.

D. repair should include the closure of visceral and parietal peritoneum to reduce postoperative adhesion formation.

E. performed electively under regional anaesthesia is as safe for the mother as normal vaginal delivery.

56. Cardiac arrest in the pregnant patient:

A. is more likely to have a successful outcome than in the non-pregnant.

B. contraindicates caesarean section.

C. may be caused by bupivacaine.

D. requires external cardiac massage in the supine position.

E. requires endotracheal intubation.

57. Spinal anaesthesia differs from epidural anaesthesia in that:

A. convulsions are more likely to result.

B. the duration of neural blockade is longer.

C. the degree of sympathetic blockade is less.

D. there is more likelihood of postdural puncture headache.

E. the onset of action of local anaesthetic is slower.

58. Postdural puncture headache:
- **A.** always presents within a few hours of inadvertent dural tap.
- **B.** is worse early in the morning.
- **C.** is relieved by paracetamol.
- **D.** is relieved by abdominal pressure.
- **E.** can be avoided by preventing straining in the second stage of labour.

59. Sensory innervation of the uterus:
- **A.** does not include any sacral contribution.
- **B.** is from the 6th to the 12th thoracic nerve roots.
- **C.** corresponds to the dermatome at the umbilicus at the upper level.
- **D.** is via the pudendal nerves.
- **E.** can be interrupted by paracervical block.

60. During general anaesthesia for caesarean section:
- **A.** failed endotracheal intubation is more likely to happen than in a general surgical patient.
- **B.** preoperative assessment is not important when there is fetal distress.
- **C.** antacid prophylaxis is important to prevent regurgitation.
- **D.** volatile anaesthetic agents provide uterine relaxation.
- **E.** blood loss is similar to that associated with regional anaesthesia.

61. Entonox:
- **A.** is a mixture of nitrous oxide and air.
- **B.** is an effective analgesic if breathed as soon as the contraction becomes painful.
- **C.** is the only approved inhalational method of analgesia.
- **D.** has a cumulative effect in a long labour.
- **E.** is a compressed gas.

62. Non-steroidal anti-inflammatory agents:
- **A.** are useful in the management of postoperative pain.
- **B.** are contraindicated in asthmatics.
- **C.** should not be used in pre-eclampsia.
- **D.** should not be used after massive haemorrhage.
- **E.** can cause gastric erosions.

63. Magnesium sulphate:

A. is the most effective anticonvulsant in preventing recurrent fits in eclampsia.
B. in a dose of 40 mg/kg attenuates the pressor response to intubation.
C. decreases the effectiveness of muscle relaxants in anaesthesia.
D. produces widespread vasodilatation and hypotension.
E. is reversed by potassium chloride.

64. In haemorrhage of pregnancy:

A. hypovolaemia is better tolerated than anaemia.
B. one should aim to restore circulating blood volume to a central venous pressure (CVP) of 5 cmH_2O.
C. for every 5 units of blood given, 2 units of fresh frozen plasma should be administered.
D. a fall in blood pressure means that a loss of at least 1500 ml of blood has occurred.
E. peripheral-core temperature difference is a useful means of determining the effectiveness of resuscitation.

65. Postdural puncture headache:

A. is characterized by a non-postural frontal or occipital headache.
B. its incidence can be lessened by the use of pencil point needles.
C. can be symptomatically relieved by intravenous caffeine.
D. can lead to auditory impairment.
E. is relieved by epidural blood patch.

66. Ambulatory or 'walking' epidurals:

A. are low-dose local anaesthetic and opiate epidural infusions.
B are a combined spinal epidural technique using local anaesthetic/opiate mixtures for both entities.
C. reduce the incidence of forceps delivery.
D. increase maternal satisfaction.
E. reduce the incidence of emergency caesarean section in labour.

67. Epidurals are indicated in labour in the following cardiovascular conditions:

A. previous myocardial infarction (MI).
B. aortic stenosis.
C. hypertrophic obstructive cardiomyopathy (HOCM).
D. Eisenmenger's syndrome.
E. Pulmonary hypertension.

68. Epidural anaesthesia is contraindicated in the following neurological diseases:

A. spina bifida occulta.
B. multiple sclerosis.
C. cerebral tumour with raised intracranial pressure.
D. myasthenia gravis.
E. epilepsy.

69. During caesarean section:

A. general anaesthesia should be avoided in those who are suxamethonium sensitive.
B. in individuals susceptible to malignant hyperthermia (MH), regional blockade is preferable to general anaesthesia.
C. both sensitivity to suxamethonium and susceptibility to malignant hyperpyrexia are inherited.
D. cricoid pressure involves approximating the thyroid cartilage to the sixth cervical vertebra and obliterating the upper oesophagus.
E. morbidity from acid aspiration can be reduced by ensuring gastric pH is above 2.5.

70. The use of low dose halogenated agents during general anaesthesia (e.g. Halothane 0.5, Isoflurane 0.75 or Enflurane 1.0%):

A. decreases maternal awareness during operation.
B. results in increased intrauterine bleeding.
C. depresses the newborn.
D. can allow 100% oxygen to be used for fetal benefit in the emergency situation.
E. probably improves uterine blood flow.

71. With regard to the use of opiates in labour:

A. pethidine is more highly protein bound in the fetus than in the mother.
B. norpethidine, a metabolite of pethidine, has a similar half-life to pethidine.
C. naloxone 0.01 mg/kg intravenously reverses the intrapartum effect of pethidine in the neonate for at least 48 hours.
D. fentanyl given epidurally can cause late respiratory depression.
E. fentanyl administered epidurally has a similar effect on gastric emptying to that of intramuscular pethidine.

72. In pre-eclampsia:

A. Swan-Ganz pulmonary artery catheterization is indicated in the presence of pulmonary oedema.
B. pulmonary oedema is associated with a CVP of 6 mmHg or more.
C. crystalloid infusions in pre-eclampsia can give rise to low oncotic pressure pulmonary oedema.
D. peripheral oxygen saturation remains normal in the presence of pulmonary oedema.
E. diuretics should be given only in the presence of an adequate circulating volume.

73. Risk factors for developing pulmonary thromboembolism in pregnancy include:

A. blood group O.
B. high parity.
C. post-term pregnancy.
D. excessive blood loss.
E. activated protein C (APC) resistance.

74. Appendicitis in pregnancy:

A. has an incidence similar to that outside pregnancy.
B. has a mortality rate similar to that outside pregnancy.
C. may be treated conservatively.
D. is more common than during the early puerperium.
E. predisposes to preterm labour.

75. In an epileptic woman who became pregnant while on valproate treatment:

A. there is a higher risk of fetal neural tube defect.
B. the risk of having a child who will develop epilepsy is 10%.
C. breastfeeding is contraindicated if the mother is still on medication during the puerperium.
D. there is a higher risk of miscarriage.
E. the one time at which seizures are more likely to occur is during or immediately after labour.

76. Vaginal delivery is contraindicated in the presence of:

A. transverse lie of the second twin.
B. central placenta praevia with a dead fetus at 28 weeks.
C. previous caesarean section for cephalopelvic disproportion.
D. cord prolapse in the second stage of labour.
E. gastroschisis.

77. Pancreatitis during pregnancy:

A. usually occurs in the first trimester.
B. is managed surgically in most cases.
C. could be safely investigated with cholangiopancreatography.
D. is associated with gallstones in over 50% of cases.
E. is associated with familial hyperlipidaemia.

78. Concerning the fetal biophysical profile (BPP) score:

A. a Doppler machine is required.
B. inclusion of fetal heart rate data improves sensitivity and specificity.
C. in the presence of acute hypoxia, fetal breathing movements are the first parameter to become abnormal.
D. has a lower false-positive rate than the non-stress test (CTG).
E. a score of 8/10 for abnormal CTG has a worse significance (i.e. higher predicted perinatal mortality) than a similar score for abnormal amniotic fluid volume.

79. When calculating the perinatal mortality rate in the UK:

A. the number of stillbirths is included in the enumerator.
B. the total number of babies dying in the neonatal period is included in the enumerator.
C. the total number of live birth is used as a denominator.
D. babies dying as a result of lethal congenital abnormality are excluded.
E. babies born dead before 28 weeks' gestation are not included.

80. Factors associated with increased perinatal mortality include:

A. primigravida.
B. high parity.
C. low birthweight.
D. increasing maternal age.
E. previous perinatal death.

81. Concerning the perinatal mortality rate in the UK:

A. the fall in the past 20 years has been largely due to improved obstetric care.
B. there are marked regional variations largely owing to differences in low birthweight.
C. ultrasonographic screening for fetal anomalies has made a significant impact in the past few years.
D. unexplained antepartum deaths constitute one-third of all perinatal deaths.
E. it is calculated per 1000 live births.

82. Regarding birthweight:

A. at term it is a good predictor of perinatal outcome.
B. low birthweight alone is a better predictor of perinatal outcome than gestational age.
C. using a cut-off of 2.5 kg at term, IUGR can be reliably detected postnatally.
D. it increases linearly to term in uncompromised pregnancies.
E. the most important determinant of birthweight is maternal weight at booking.

83. In rubella infection:
- **A.** the mode of transmission is faeco-oral.
- **B.** the period of infectivity is from 7 days before to 7 days after the appearance of the rash.
- **C.** the diagnosis is usually made by viral isolation.
- **D.** it can take up to 21 days after exposure for specific IgM to appear in the blood.
- **E.** specific IgM persists in the blood for 6 months.

84. Human parvovirus B19 infection during pregnancy:
- **A.** is usually asymptomatic.
- **B.** is a recognized cause of haemolytic anaemia in the fetus.
- **C.** should be considered in the differential of a low maternal serum α-fetoprotein (AFP) levels.
- **D.** is associated with congenital abnormality.
- **E.** is a recognized cause of aplastic anaemia in the mother.

85. The lupus anticoagulant:
- **A.** is present in about 10% of the obstetric population.
- **B.** may be associated with a fetal loss rate in excess of 50%.
- **C.** causes prolongation of the clotting time in vitro.
- **D.** results in an increased risk of thrombosis.
- **E.** is a recognized cause of congenital heart block.

86. Recognized maternal risk factors for pre-eclampsia include:
- **A.** pre-eclampsia in a previous pregnancy.
- **B.** high social class.
- **C.** teenage.
- **D.** family history of pre-eclampsia.
- **E.** obesity.

87. Maternal mortality:
- **A.** according to the International Classification of Diseases – ninth revision (ICD9) includes deaths up to 42 days after the termination of pregnancy.
- **B.** includes fortuitous deaths.
- **C.** includes direct and indirect deaths.
- **D.** in the UK accounts for less than 1% of deaths in women aged 15–44 years.
- **E.** amounts to half a million mothers or mothers-to-be in the world every year.

88. With regard to Confidential Enquiries into Maternal Deaths:

A. the responsibility for initiating the enquiries rests with the doctor who signs the death certificate.
B. the first UK report covered the years 1952–1954.
C. the Coroner is involved.
D. confidentiality is paramount.
E. there is a Regional Midwife Assessor.

89. With regard to Confidential Enquiries into Maternal Deaths:

A. English death certificates contain a specific question on pregnancy.
B. fortuitous deaths are due to a cause not related to or influenced by pregnancy.
C. deaths more than 42 days after termination are excluded.
D. substandard care is the term used for an avoidable death.
E. more than 95% of known maternal deaths are investigated by the enquiries.

90. In the Report on Confidential Enquiries into Maternal Deaths in the UK 1991–1993:

A. the risk of death increased with maternal age.
B. the main cause of direct death was pulmonary embolism.
C. there was substandard care in more than half the deaths from hypertensive diseases of pregnancy.
D. there were more direct deaths associated with planned emergency than with unplanned emergency caesarean section.
E. more women died from illegal than from legal abortion.

91. Listeriosis:

A. can be diagnosed by blood culture.
B. occurs exclusively in the third trimester.
C. causes intrauterine death.
D. can be treated with ampicillin.
E. has a predilection for immunocompromised individuals.

92. In the Report on Confidential Enquiries into Maternal Deaths in the UK 1988–1990:

A. most postpartum direct deaths from pulmonary embolism occurred following caesarean section.
B. there was a decrease in deaths associated with genital tract sepsis.
C. 11% of direct deaths were associated with anaesthesia.
D. recommendations were made that evacuated uterine contents need not be sent for histological examination.
E. autopsy was carried out in over four-fifths of all deaths.

93. In diabetes mellitus:

A. corticosteroids should be given before delivery if it is anticipated before 32 weeks .
B. ritodrine to suppress preterm labour is contraindicated.
C. periconceptional folic acid should be prescribed.
D. the combined oral contraceptive pill is not advised.
E. the failure rate of the coil (intrauterine contraceptive device; IUCD) is greater than in non-diabetics.

94. In a pregnant woman with diabetes mellitus:

A. the incidence of major malformation is increased when the HbA_1C is greater than 10% at 16 weeks.
B. the incidence of cardiac anomalies is increased.
C. anencephaly is more common.
D. spontaneous abortion is more common with poor early glycaemic control.
E. there is an early growth delay between conception and 7 weeks.

95. The infant of a diabetic mother has an increased risk of:

A. neonatal jaundice.
B. macrocytic anaemia.
C. hypokalaemia.
D. cardiomegaly.
E. Erb's palsy.

96. A glucose tolerance test (GTT) should be done in pregnancy when:

A. a previous male baby weighed more than 4000 g at 42 weeks.
B. there is a history of previous shoulder dystocia.
C. unexplained polyhydramnios develops.
D. the mother's weight is 103 kg.
E. there is insulin-dependent diabetes in the partner's family.

97. In gestational diabetes (glucose intolerance first recognized in pregnancy):

A. the prevalence is increased in Asians.
B. one in eight develop insulin-dependent diabetes within 5 years.
C. obesity is a risk factor.
D. the prevalence is increased in Afro-Caribbeans.
E. the congenital malformation rate is increased.

98. Concerning shoulder dystocia:

A. previous shoulder dystocia is a predictor.
B. the incidence increases with prolonged second stage.
C. ultrasonography gives an accurate fetal weight estimation.
D. the McRoberts position should be adopted.
E. suprapubic pressure is used in management.

99. The fetal biophysical profile (BPP) score:

A. may be unreliable under 26 weeks' gestation.
B. requires continuous fetal breathing for at least 60 seconds for a full score (10/10).
C. accounts for the presence of abnormally increased amniotic fluid volume.
D. is usually based on a score of 0 or 2 for each factor but intermediate scores of 1 may be awarded in some circumstances.
E. assumes the fetus is neurologically normal.

100. With regard to Doppler ultrasonographic equipment:

A. pulsed-wave devices may be used to calculate blood velocity.

B. pulsed-wave devices may be used to calculate blood flow.

C. a low-pass filter is used to remove artefact from vessel wall motion.

D. continuous-wave devices may be used to calculate blood velocity.

E. continuous-wave devices may be used to calculate blood flow.

101. Umbilical artery waveform indices:

A. correlate well with spiral artery count.

B. correlate well with tertiary stem villi count.

C. correlate well with short-term morbidity in high-risk pregnancy.

D. correlate well with long-term outcome in high-risk pregnancy.

E. are discordant in twin–twin transfusion syndrome.

102. Uteroplacental Doppler waveforms:

A. exhibit notching in pregnancies at risk of pre-eclampsia.

B. exhibit notching in pregnancies at risk of intrauterine growth retardation.

C. exhibit notching in pregnancies at risk of hypoxia.

D. exhibit a reduction in Pulsatility Index in normal pregnancy.

E. may be reliably assessed using continuous-wave Doppler devices.

103. Absent end-diastolic velocity in the umbilical artery waveform:

A. implies a high risk of fetal death in utero.

B. the wall thump filter should be less than 100 Hz.

C. progression to reversed end-diastolic velocities implies worsening fetal condition.

D. is not associated with an increased risk of structural abnormalities.

E. is not associated with an increased risk of chromosomal abnormalities.

104. Absent end-diastolic velocity in the umbilical artery waveform:
- **A.** should prompt delivery if the fetus is viable.
- **B.** should prompt intensive fetal surveillance.
- **C.** should be followed by delivery only for non-Doppler indications.
- **D.** implies a Resistance Index (RI) of 1.0.
- **E.** is found in about 5% of fetuses at 34 weeks.

105. Regarding colour Doppler ultrasonography:
- **A.** blue is used to denote venous flow.
- **B.** red denotes flow away from the transducer.
- **C.** brightness relates to flow velocity.
- **D.** it improves the diagnosis of congenital heart disease.
- **E.** it may be of value in diagnosing renal agenesis.

106. Concerning power Doppler ultrasonography:
- **A.** brightness is related to amplitude.
- **B.** direction of flow is indicated by changes in colour.
- **C.** sensitivity is greater for detection of low-velocity flow compared with colour Doppler ultrasonography.
- **D.** aliasing is reduced.
- **E.** enables identification of redistribution of fetal blood flow in hypoxia.

107. Concerning the safety of Doppler ultrasonsography:
- **A.** colour Doppler ultrasonography exposes the fetus to higher doses of ultrasound than pulse-wave Doppler imaging.
- **B.** cavitation, microbubble formation and heating may occur at the bone-soft tissue interfaces along the pulsed-wave Doppler beam.
- **C.** cavitation, microbubble formation and heating may occur at the bone-soft tissue interfaces, maximally in the area delineated by the sample gate of the pulsed-wave Doppler beam.
- **D.** heating of about 1°C may occur at bone-soft tissue interfaces with conventional obstetric pulsed-wave Doppler ultrasonography.
- **E.** intensively scanned fetuses have lower birthweights than those exposed to minimum imaging and Doppler ultrasonography in utero.

108. Regarding umbilical artery waveform indices:

A. Pulsatility Index can be measured when end-diastolic velocities are absent or reversed.

B. Resistance Index is zero when end-diastolic velocities are absent or reversed.

C. the greater the Pulsatility Index, the higher the implied placental vascular impedance.

D. the measurements are independent of the angle of insonation.

E. they are dimensionless.

109. In ultrasonographic fetal biometry:

A. an abdominal circumference (AC) measurement less than the fifth centile is diagnostic of intrauterine growth restriction (IUGR).

B. an abnormally high head circumference/abdominal circumference ratio (HC/AC) in a small for gestational age (SGA) fetus is more likely to be the result of uteroplacental insufficiency than of a chromosomal abnormality.

C. weekly biometry is valuable in monitoring growth in pregnancies at risk of IUGR.

D. abdominal circumference measurements indirectly reflect fetal liver size and glycogen storage.

E. serial biparietal diameter (BPD) measurements are an important part of third trimester monitoring in IUGR pregnancies.

110. Regarding ultrasonographic fetal biometry:

A. in late pregnancy the femur length/abdominal circumference (FL/AC) ratio is useful in determining the aetiology of intrauterine growth restriction (IUGR).

B. classical type I or symmetrical IUGR may be due to chromosomal abnormality or fetal infection.

C. classical type I or symmetrical IUGR may be constitutional or ethnic in origin

D. correction should be made for maternal factors such as height, weight, parity and ethnic background.

E. the AC measurement should be made at the level of the fetal stomach and liver.

111. Regarding ultrasonographic fetal biometry:
- **A.** discordant head circumference in twin pregnancy may indicate twin–twin transfusion syndrome.
- **B.** a single ultrasonographic scan at 32 weeks has an 85% detection rate for subsequent delivery of a small for dates baby.
- **C.** estimated fetal weight is accurate to about ±5% in the third trimester.
- **D.** linear measurements such as femur length are accurate to about ±2% in the third trimester.
- **E.** suspected fetal macrosomia can be excluded by a careful ultrasonographic scan and subsequent estimation of fetal weight.

112. Regarding maternally perceived fetal movements:
- **A.** in the third trimester one would usually expect at least ten movements by 1800 hours.
- **B.** routine use of kick charts in low-risk pregnancies has been shown to reduce perinatal mortality.
- **C.** the false-positive rate of kick charts is high for perinatal mortality.
- **D.** in the third trimester an anterior placenta may mask the maternal appreciation of fetal movements.
- **E.** fetal activity is reduced at term in normal fetuses.

113. In the FIGO definitions of antenatal cardiotocography:
- **A.** a normal baseline should be 120–160 bpm.
- **B.** normal amplitude of baseline variability should be 5–25 bpm.
- **C.** normally two or more accelerations should be present in 20 minutes.
- **D.** maternally perceived fetal movements should normally be associated with accelerations.
- **E.** recurrent late decelerations are classified as suspicious.

114. Late decelerations on an intrapartum fetal cardiotocogram are commoner in:
- **A.** rhesus disease.
- **B.** maternal renal disease.
- **C.** IUGR.
- **D.** antiphospholipid antibody syndrome.
- **E.** diabetes mellitus.

115. Management of late decelerations on an intrapartum fetal cardiotocogram should include:
A. change in maternal position.
B. stopping oxytocics.
C. checking maternal blood pressure.
D. fetal blood sampling if variability is also reduced.
E. delivery if there is a baseline tachycardia.

116. Regarding antenatal fetal heart rate tracing:
A. the oxytocin challenge test carries significant risks to the fetus and should be carried out only when patients are fully fasted and prepared for caesarean section.
B. a reactive non-stress test is defined as two accelerations of more than 15 bpm and of 15 seconds' duration in 20 min.
C. an abnormal non-stress test is one in which the above criteria are not met in 40 minutes.
D. the false-negative rate is of the non-stress test is 3.2 per 1000 (fetal death in 24 hours).
E. the false-positive rate of the non-stress test is 10%.

117. Current indications for amniocentesis include:
A. maternal age over 35 years.
B. a Down's syndrome risk of 1 in 128 on serum testing.
C. raised maternal serum α-fetoprotein of more than 2.2 multiples of the median.
D. gross obesity in a women with a previous child with spina bifida.
E. mild to moderate rhesus disease.

118. Recognized complications of prenatal invasive diagnostic tests include:
A. a miscarriage risk of 5% for amniocentesis.
B. a risk of limb reduction defects for chorionic villus sampling (CVS) performed before 10 weeks.
C. a risk of neonatal postural limb defects following amniocentesis.
D. an increased risk of miscarriage if amniocentesis is performed at 13 rather than 16 weeks.
E. rhesus isoimmunization in rhesus-negative women.

119. Antenatal fetal blood sampling:

A. should be performed under continuous ultrasonographic guidance.
B. should not be performed before 18–20 weeks' gestation.
C. may lead to fetal cord tamponade.
D. is always performed through the umbilical vein.
E. is a recognized indication in IUGR pregnancies.

120. Coccygodynia:

A. is caused by childbirth.
B. is treated by coccygectomy.
C. pain is referred to the upper vagina.
D. may be exacerbated by defaecation.
E. may be exacerbated by micturition.

121. In multiple pregnancy:

A. scanning should be arranged at 20 weeks to assess the zygosity.
B. fetuses of similar sex are monozygotic.
C. scanning in the first trimester can assess fetal number and chorionicity.
D. a membrane detected on ultrasonography indicates a dichorionic pregnancy.
E. fetuses of disparate sex indicate dizygotic twins.

122. A raised maternal serum α-fetoprotein (AFP) level is found in association with:

A. recent fetal demise.
B. Dandy-Walker malformation.
C. recent amniocentesis.
D. fetal multicystic kidney.
E. an omphalocele.

123. In a pregnancy with fetal neural tube defect:

A. the maternal α-fetoprotein (AFP) level is always raised.
B. greater than 90% of cases show an abnormality in the head.
C. fetal lower limb movement is a good predictor of outcome.
D. the cerebellum is normal in 50% of cases.
E. the level of the lesion predicts outcome.

124. The following ultrasonographic findings are associated with an increased incidence of chromosomal abnormality:

A. facial clefts.
B. nuchal translucency greater than 3 mm at 10–13 weeks' gestation.
C. jejunal atresia.
D. diaphragmatic hernia.
E. tracheo-oesophageal fistula.

125. A rhesus-negative multigravida who has had one previous caesarean section presents at 34 weeks' gestation with vaginal bleeding. The following statements are correct:

A. Transvaginal ultrasonography is contraindicated.
B. The presence of a fundal placenta excludes the diagnosis of placenta praevia.
C. If, on ultrasonography, the leading edge of the placenta lies 6 cm from the internal os, vaginal delivery is not contraindicated.
D. If the Kleihauer test is negative, she should not receive anti-D immunoglobulins.
E. The diagnosis of placental abruption can be excluded by a normal ultrasonographic examination.

126. Fetal breathing movements:

A. increase within 48 hours of the onset of labour.
B. are associated with the passage of meconium.
C. may be reduced in fetal hypoxia.
D. are primarily due to the movements of the intercostal muscles.
E. are associated with gaseous exchange within the lungs.

127. Iron deficiency anaemia in pregnancy is associated with a reduction in:

A. mean red cell volume.
B. serum iron concentration.
C. total iron-binding capacity.
D. haemoglobin concentration.
E. mean red cell haemoglobin.

128. α-Fetoprotein:

A. is a glycoprotein.
B. is produced in the yolk sac.
C. reaches its highest concentration in the maternal serum at about 16 weeks' gestation.
D. has a similar concentration in fetal serum and amniotic fluid.
E. shows an abnormally reduced concentration in second-trimester maternal serum in cases of Down's syndrome (47,+21).

129. Normal changes in the electrocardiogram during pregnancy include:

A. deviation of the electrical axis to the left.
B. a loud third heart sound.
C. Q wave in lead III.
D. shortened P-R interval.
E. increased rate.

130. During intrauterine life:

A. the male fetus grows at a higher rate than the female fetus from the 28th week of gestation.
B. the placenta grows at a slower rate than the fetus during the third trimester.
C. the lungs are not capable of exchanging gases sufficient to support life before the 28th week of gestation.
D. fetal blood glucose levels are higher than those of the mother.
E. fetal arterial pressure increases throughout pregnancy.

131. During the second trimester of normal pregnancy there is a progressive increase in the production of:

A. human chorionic gonadotrophin.
B. oestriol.
C. human placental lactogen.
D. luteinizing hormone.
E. progesterone.

132. Oxytocin:

A. is a nonapeptide.
B. is synthesized in the posterior lobe of the pituitary gland.
C. receptor concentration in the uterus increases towards the end of pregnancy.
D. secretion is stimulated by alcohol.
E. has some antidiuretic action.

133. Lactation:

A. is initiated postnatally in response to the rising levels of oestrogen.
B. does not occur in the absence of maternal pituitary growth hormone.
C. can inhibit ovulation.
D. is inhibited by progesterone.
E. is inhibited by bromocriptine.

134. An antenatal screening test for pre-eclampsia was evaluated in 100 primigravid women; 20 were screen-positive. At the end of the study only ten women developed pre-eclampsia; only five of them were of the 20 screen-positive women. The:

A. sensitivity of the test is 50%.
B. specificity of the test is 10%.
C. positive predictive value of the test is 25%.
D. negative predictive value of the test is 5%.
E. test would be expected to have similar performance if applied to the whole pregnant population (primigravid and multigravid).

135. Drugs contraindicated during breastfeeding include:

A. warfarin.
B. methyldopa.
C. penicillin.
D. metronidazole.
E. carbamazepine.

136. Methyldopa:

A. acts mainly on the peripheral α-adrenergic receptors.
B. can cause a positive direct antiglobulin (Coombs) test.
C. is a fast-acting hypotensive agent.
D. can cause depression.
E. can cause haemolytic anaemia.

137. Side-effects of oxytocin include:
- **A.** fetal distress.
- **B.** hypernatraemia.
- **C.** amniotic fluid embolism.
- **D.** uterine rupture.
- **E.** hyperprolactinaemia.

138. Drugs that are teratogenic in the human include:
- **A.** bromocriptine.
- **B.** methyldopa.
- **C.** metronidazole.
- **D.** carbamazepine.
- **E.** diethylstilboestrol.

139. External cephalic version (ECV) of breech:
- **A.** should not be carried out after 37 weeks' gestation.
- **B.** is associated with an increased risk of placental abruption.
- **C.** is associated with about a 1% risk of fetal mortality.
- **D.** can significantly reduce the incidence of caesarean section.
- **E.** should ideally be performed under general anaesthesia.

140. Monozygotic twinning:
- **A.** is associated with single chorion, amnion and placenta in only 1% of cases.
- **B.** is associated with higher complications compared with dizygotic twinning.
- **C.** has a higher incidence among Europeans.
- **D.** is associated with a 10% risk of conjoined twins.
- **E.** is associated with an increased incidence of fetal anomalies.

141. Postoperative haemorrhage in caesarean hysterectomy:
- **A.** in the majority of cases occurs within the first 48 hours.
- **B.** commonly occurs as a result of a vascular pedicle becoming freed from its ligature.
- **C.** is usually obvious as vaginal bleeding.
- **D.** is more common following intraoperative haemorrhage.
- **E.** can be caused by coagulopathy.

142. Recognized risk factors in infection following caesarean section include:

A. long duration of labour regardless of the condition of the membranes.
B. rupture of the membranes.
C. epidural anaesthesia.
D. internal electronic fetal heart rate monitoring.
E. obesity.

143. Erb's palsy in the neonate is:

A. usually self-limiting with complete recovery.
B. a particular hazard in shoulder dystocia.
C. a result of trauma to the lower part of the brachial plexus.
D. associated with possible diaphragmatic paralysis.
E. an indication for early surgical intervention.

144. Neonatal conjugated hyperbilirubinaemia is:

A. the common form of neonatal physiological jaundice.
B. associated with the passage of bilirubin in the urine.
C. a possible manifestation of galactosaemia.
D. a common feature in very bruised babies.
E. an indication to perform diagnostic tests for biliary atresia.

145. In neonatal resuscitation:

A. drugs are the mainstay of management.
B. the Apgar score at 1 minute is useful in determining long-term prognosis.
C. the Apgar score at 10 minutes is useful in determining long-term progress.
D. passive inflations are pressure-regulated to reduce the possibility of air leak.
E. suspicion of meconium in major airways is an indication to avoid 'bag and mask' ventilation.

146. Breastfeeding success can be increased by:
- **A.** helping mothers initiate breastfeeding within half an hour of birth.
- **B.** rooming-in mothers and infants together 24 hours a day.
- **C.** avoiding artificial pacifiers (soothers) for breastfeeding infants.
- **D.** encouraging breastfeeding on demand.
- **E.** complementing breastfeeds with dextrose or formula in hungry babies.

147. The following groups of babies are at increased risk of hypoglycaemia:
- **A.** hypothermia after delivery.
- **B.** congenital infection.
- **C.** birth asphyxia.
- **D.** respiratory distress syndrome.
- **E.** appropriately grown post-term infant (3.9 kg).

148. Respiratory distress syndrome in preterm babies is:
- **A.** more likely in babies delivered by caesarean section.
- **B.** reduced in incidence by antenatal steroid administration.
- **C.** always evident within 12 hours of delivery.
- **D.** treatable by intravenous surfactant administration.
- **E.** still an important cause of neonatal mortality in the UK.

149. In congenital diaphragmatic hernia:
- **A.** the defect is usually right sided.
- **B.** there is an overall survival rate of over 50%.
- **C.** presentation can be as a respiratory emergency at birth.
- **D.** the condition can be asymptomatic throughout infancy.
- **E.** the main predictor of outcome is the volume of herniated organs in the chest.

150. Causes of neonatal jaundice include:
- **A.** ampicillin therapy.
- **B.** congenital toxoplasmosis.
- **C.** ABO haemolytic diseases of the newborn.
- **D.** spherocytosis.
- **E.** rhesus isoimmunization.

151. Compared with the adult, the neonate has a reduced concentration of:

A. vitamin K.
B. protein S.
C. clotting factor VIII.
D. antithrombin III.
E. clotting factor X.

152. The following are autosomal recessive conditions:

A. Duchenne muscular dystrophy.
B. achondroplasia.
C. infantile polycystic renal disease.
D. Huntington's disease.
E. Fallot's tetralogy.

153. The following are at risk of developing haemophilia:

A. a male child with an affected father.
B. a male child with an affected cousin on his mother's side.
C. a girl with Turner's syndrome whose mother is a carrier of haemophilia.
D. a boy with Down's syndrome due to a 14/21 translocation.
E. a girl whose mother is a carrier and whose father is affected.

154. Autosomal recessive conditions include:

A. Huntington's disease.
B. Meckel-Gruber syndrome.
C. Joubert's syndrome.
D. achondroplasia.
E. cystic fibrosis.

155. Triploidy:

A. is typically associated with young paternal age.
B. is commonly found in live-born children with multiple abnormalities.
C. is caused by three sets of haploid chromosomes.
D. is typically associated with severe intrauterine growth restriction (IUGR).
E. can manifest as a partial hydatidiform mole.

156. Prenatal diagnosis for a recessive disease by gene tracking:
A. requires DNA from an affected child.
B. is available for all recessive diseases.
C. is optimally undertaken at the gestational age at which the gene is expressed.
D. carries a low error rate if the DNA markers are widely spaced.
E. is best organized through a family study.

157. DNA diagnosis for a dominant condition (such as Marfan's syndrome):
A. will be highly accurate if the familial mutation has been identified.
B. usually requires a family history to determine linkage phase if DNA markers and gene tracking are to be used.
C. may not be possible if DNA markers are uninformative.
D. may give an inaccurate result if there is genetic heterogeneity.
E. can be useful in cases with equivocal clinical signs.

158. An additional chromosome marker found on fetal karyotyping:
A. is an absolute indication for recommending termination of pregnancy.
B. is unlikely to cause clinical effects if present in a normal parent.
C. carries a better prognosis the smaller its size.
D. requires further investigations to determine its chromosome of origin.
E. will cause no clinical effects if structural malformations are not detected on ultrasonography.

159. A culture of cells obtained at chorionic villus sampling showed two populations: one containing the normal chromosome complement, the other containing an additional chromosome. The chromosomal mosaicism:

A. may be due to contamination by maternal cells.
B. may be caused by confined placental mosaicism.
C. in this case should be confirmed by karyotyping cells obtained by amniocentesis or fetal blood sampling.
D. is likely to cause minimal effects on the fetus as normal cells are also present.
E. is less likely to be due to a cultural artefact if found in several cultures.

160. When the fetal karyotype 47,XYY is found at amniocentesis, the parents should be told that:

A. the boy will be infertile.
B. his physical appearance will be normal.
C. there is a 30% chance that gynaecomastia will develop.
D. severe mental retardation would not be expected.
E. the recurrence risk increases with increasing maternal age.

161. Chromosome analysis is indicated in a:

A. fetus with multiple congenital abnormalities.
B. child presenting with retinoblastoma.
C. couple who have had four early pregnancy losses.
D. neonate with ambiguous genitalia.
E. couple with a previous baby with a neural tube defect.

162. A man is the only person in his family affected with a genetic condition which was diagnosed at the age of 19 years. The clinician can assume he has a negligible risk of having a similarly affected child if his diagnosis is:

A. retinitis pigmentosa.
B. polycystic kidney disease.
C. hypercholesterolaemia.
D. bilateral cataracts.
E. sensorineural deafness.

163. Genetic counselling:
- **A.** should give the patient a clear outline of all the options available.
- **B.** is a communication process dealing with the risk of developing and transmitting a genetic condition.
- **C.** has as its main purpose the reduction in genetic disease in the population.
- **D.** is best undertaken before pregnancy is planned.
- **E.** is not necessary if the risk is less than 1 in 4.

164. A detailed family history is useful:
- **A.** in determining the most appropriate prenatal diagnostic investigations which could be offered.
- **B.** in identifying most couples at risk of having babies with multiple congenital anomalies.
- **C.** in identifying couples at a higher risk of autosomal recessive disorders.
- **D.** in reassuring couples in cousin marriages they are not at increased risk of having a child with a genetic disease.
- **E.** for calculating carrier risks for females in X-linked disorders.

165. Carriers of a balanced reciprocal chromosome translocation:
- **A.** have a high incidence of minor physical anomalies.
- **B.** are the result of a *de novo* event in most cases.
- **C.** usually have 46 chromosomes.
- **D.** usually have a chromosomal rearrangement unique to their family.
- **E.** are found in the general population with an incidence of approximately 1 in 500.

166. A girl with normal external genitalia was born following amniocentesis for maternal age which had predicted that the baby would be male. A likely cause requiring further investigation is that the baby has:
- **A.** congenital adrenal hyperplasia.
- **B.** testicular feminization syndrome.
- **C.** Turner's syndrome.
- **D.** 45,X/46,XY mosaicism.
- **E.** true hermaphroditism.

167. The sister of a boy with Duchenne muscular dystrophy presented in the 11th week of pregnancy. Her brother is the only known person with muscular dystrophy in the family. She:

A. is at a very low risk of being a carrier.
B. could be offered definitive prenatal diagnosis by chorionic villus sampling if her brother was found to have a deletion of the dystrophic gene.
C. should have her carrier status checked by creatine kinase estimation immediately.
D. should be referred for an urgent genetic opinion.
E. will require no further investigations during this pregnancy to determine fetal status if the fetus is a female.

168. A patient comments at her first antenatal clinic visit at 9 weeks that her partner had a sister who died with cystic fibrosis as a child 20 years ago. As part of the offer of DNA testing, she should be told that:

A. there is a risk of 2 out of 3 that her partner is a carrier.
B. her baby would have a 1 in 4 risk of being affected if both she and her partner were carriers.
C. both she and her partner can be tested for the common mutations of the cystic fibrosis gene.
D. there would be a small residual risk of their having an affected child if neither of them was shown to have any of the common mutations.
E. accurate prenatal diagnosis would be possible if a mutation was identified in both of them.

169. A family had a rare structural anomaly of the hands, inherited in a dominant pattern. A girl with the anomaly was born to a man with apparently normal hands. His father, sister and two brothers had the anomaly. An affected child being born to an unaffected parent could be due to:

A. variation in expression.
B. lack of penetrance.
C. a new mutation.
D. a phenocopy.
E. mistaken paternity.

170. Conditions with autosomal dominant inheritance include:
- **A.** galactosaemia.
- **B.** multiple neurofibromatosis.
- **C.** haemophilia.
- **D.** tuberose sclerosis.
- **E.** osteogenesis imperfecta.

171. Nuclear chromatin (Barr body):
- **A.** represents an inactivated X chromosome that could be of paternal origin.
- **B.** is present in androgen insensitivity syndrome.
- **C.** is observed during interphase.
- **D.** does not appear in the cells of the normal female embryo until the ovaries have developed.
- **E.** is present in female Down's syndrome (trisomy 21).

172. Regarding Turner's syndrome (45,X):
- **A.** there is only one nuclear chromatin (Barr body).
- **B.** there is an increased risk of spontaneous abortion in affected embryos.
- **C.** there is increased incidence with increased maternal age.
- **D.** no germ cells are present during intrauterine development.
- **E.** short stature is a phenotypic feature.

173. An individual with the karyotype 46,XX t (X;7) (p21;q23) will have:
- **A.** a female phenotype.
- **B.** a normal number of chromosomes.
- **C.** a translocation involving the long arm of the X chromosome.
- **D.** a translocation involving band 7 of the X chromosome.
- **E.** increased risk of reproductive loss.

174. An individual with trisomy 21 (47,XX,+21):
- **A.** can produce chromosomally normal children.
- **B.** usually has an IQ of 25–50.
- **C.** has an increased likelihood of Hirschsprung's disease.
- **D.** has an increased likelihood of acute leukaemia.
- **E.** may result from chromosomal translocation.

175. In a balanced chromosomal reciprocal translocation carrier there is:
- **A.** normal number of chromosomes.
- **B.** normal amount of genetic material.
- **C.** normal arrangement of genetic material.
- **D.** increased risk of reproductive loss.
- **E.** greater risk of cytogenetically abnormal offspring if the carrier is a female rather than male.

176. Breech presentation at the onset of labour is associated with:
- **A.** prematurity.
- **B.** placenta praevia.
- **C.** cornual placenta.
- **D.** full maternal bladder.
- **E.** breech presentation at term in a previous pregnancy.

177. Face presentation in labour is associated with:
- **A.** post-term pregnancy.
- **B.** anencephaly.
- **C.** dolichocephaly.
- **D.** fetal goitre.
- **E.** an incidence of about 1 in 500.

178. In cases of transverse lie:
- **A.** there is associated placenta praevia in about 10% of cases.
- **B.** arm prolapse is more common than cord prolapse.
- **C.** the fetal back is usually anterior.
- **D.** the fetal head is commonly to the mother's left.
- **E.** of the second twin, caesarean section is the treatment of choice.

179. With regard to rubella:
- **A.** if a woman was tested and found to be immune in a previous pregnancy, she need not have another test in subsequent pregnancies.
- **B.** maternal infection in the first trimester is associated with an affected fetus in almost all cases.
- **C.** IgM takes up to 21 days to appear in the blood after infection.
- **D.** there is no risk to the fetus from rubella immunization during pregnancy.
- **E.** reinfection after previous immunization can occur.

180. Secondary postpartum haemorrhage:

A. most commonly occurs during the first postpartum week.
B. could be due to choriocarcinoma.
C. should be treated by evacuation of the uterus based on an ultrasonographic examination suggestive of retained products of conception.
D. may present with a life-threatening haemorrhage following caesarean delivery.
E. is reduced in incidence by a policy of active management of the third stage of labour.

181. Intrahepatic cholestasis of pregnancy is associated with:

A. preterm labour.
B. intrauterine fetal death.
C. low levels of bile acids.
D. pruritus, typically in the second trimester.
E. marked geographical variation in incidence.

182. Women who develop the following conditions during their first pregnancy are at a higher risk of recurrence in subsequent pregnancies compared with matched controls:

A. pre-eclampsia.
B. cholestasis of pregnancy.
C. preterm labour.
D. placenta praevia.
E. placental abruption.

183. With regard to imaging techniques during pregnancy:

A. Doppler ultrasonography can exclude iliac vein thrombosis.
B. a radiographic contrast venogram exposes the fetus to a radiation dose of about 0.5 rad.
C. computed tomographic (CT) pelvimetry exposes the fetus to more radiation than radiographic pelvimetry.
D. V/Q scanning should not be performed during the first trimester.
E. a V/Q scan exposes the fetus to more radiation than a radiographic contrast venogram.

Answers

1. AD

'HELLP' is an acronym which stands for *H*aemolysis, *E*levated *L*iver enzymes, *L*ow *P*latelets and was originally described by Weinstein in 1982. However, usually in pregnancy the *H* represents hypertension. The severity of the condition has been divided on the basis of the platelet count into Class 1 < 50,000/mm^3, Class 2 50,000–100,000/mm^3 and Class 3 100,000–150,000/mm^3. The liver enzymes, namely the transaminases, are those that are raised and represent the degree of liver damage that exists. The alkaline phosphatase concentration is not raised specifically in HELLP but may become so in the presence of extensive, and probably terminal, obstructive liver damage. Eclampsia is a fairly common feature of HELLP, leading to the probability that they are part of the same disease process. HELLP recurs in about 60% of pregnancies when it occurs in the index pregnancy before 32 weeks. If after 32 weeks, a recurrence rate of around 10% is found.

2. B

Maternal cardiac output rises rapidly in the first trimester of pregnancy so that substantial increases have occurred by about 13–14 weeks. Overall cardiac output increases about 40–50% before labour starts with further increases once in labour. In the first stage cardiac output may rise to 8–10 litres and in an active second stage to as high as 14 litres. Cardiac output can be controlled, not enhanced, by adequate pain relief through epidural anaesthesia, and the peripheral vasodilatation can be used to modify the volume of blood returning to the heart. Regardless of the cardiac lesion, cardiac output increases during the second stage of labour. Cardiac output takes some time to return to pre-pregnancy levels but will have done so by 4–6 weeks after delivery.

3. AC

Studies concerning the sensitivity of ultrasonography for the detection of neural tube defects suggest a figure close to 100% compared with about 85% using maternal serum AFP screening. On the other hand, routine scanning for cardiac anomalies seems less successful, with even good units reporting 50–60% detection rates; some detection rates are as low as 4%.

Ultrasonography to detect placental site up to 20 weeks is unreliable and will tend to overcall. The incidence of placenta praevia at term is similar in women who have a low-lying placenta on scan at 20 weeks and in those who do not, and many units are moving away from routinely rescanning the former.

The first trimester, perhaps 11–12 weeks, is the best time to assess chorionicity in twins. Of course, sexing at 20 weeks is possible and, if different, is pretty conclusive! The current thinking on choroid plexus cysts is that, in isolation, they may indicate an overall risk of trisomy 18 of about 1 in 150 and about 1 in 800 for trisomy 21.

4. A

Nephrotic syndrome is defined as a condition associated with a urinary protein loss of 3 g per day and a serum albumin concentration of less than 30 g per litre. The condition arises in the presence of extensive renal damage, usually glomerular or tubular. In the case of renal vein thrombosis, changes probably occur as the result of back pressure. None of the other conditions listed is associated with nephrotic syndrome. Kidney stones may be associated with some proteinuria but this is not extensive. Polycystic renal disease may also be associated with some proteinuria, whereas essential hypertension is used only to describe unexplained hypertension. The antiphospholipid syndrome is not associated with renal damage.

5. BCDE

Diabetes can confuse the information derived from the BPP because there may be a falsely reassuring amount of amniotic fluid present, amniotic fluid volume being the component with the highest predictive value. Thus the warning that all may not be well, which often comes from reduced amounts of amniotic fluid, will be lost.

The BPP allows evaluation of each baby in multiple pregnancies and is preferable than the cardiotocography (CTG) alone. The BPP was originally devised to assess the post-dates pregnancy. Fetal condition is an important assessment in maternal hypertensive disease. However, the original concept that a normal BPP implies that the baby would be unlikely to die within 1 week did not hold in the presence of intrauterine growth restriction, so care must be taken in the evaluation of such babies when the mother has hypertension.

The BPP in the presence of ruptured membranes is generally considered of use but, of course, there is no useful information to be gained from amniotic fluid measurements. On the other hand the presence of fetal breathing movements makes intrauterine infection unlikely.

6. C

Fetal abnormality is now the number one killer in diabetes. Most data suggest that the pregnancy-related diabetic nephropathy improves following delivery. Caesarean section remains high in diabetes. IUGR does not correlate with HbA_1C. It does, however, correlate with the duration of diabetes, especially if this extends past 20 years. Although caudal regression syndrome seems to be specific to diabetes it is extremely rare – cardiac and central nervous system anomalies are the commonest.

7. DE

Prophylaxis postpartum in adequate doses is effective in all but about 1% of cases. A maternal serum antibody level of greater than 4 iu/ml is an indication for amniocentesis. The amniotic fluid is examined at three wavelengths: 385, 450 and 550 A. PCR can now be used to assess fetal Rh status with a good degree of accuracy. Maternal prophylaxis at 28 and 34 weeks is an effective way of preventing sensitization; what is less clear is whether it is cost effective.

8. AD

In general, measurements made after 26 weeks tend to be unreliable for dating. The head/trunk ratio is not helpful mainly because of the difficulties of making accurate trunk measurements at this time and the fact that the ratio does not give specific dating information. Gestation sac diameter is of greater use in very early pregnancy up to about 8 weeks, when it measures about 30 mm.

9. BCE

Hydralazine has a direct effect on vasculature not mediated by calcium channels. Methyldopa does have a depressing effect. Atenolol has been shown to be associated with IUGR but only when used in essential hypertension. Women with 'chronic hypertension' on atenolol should have their antihypertensive changed if possible when planning a pregnancy or early in its course. Angiotensin-converting enzyme (ACE) inhibitors are not safe in pregnancy and have possible teratogenic effects, and have been associated with IUGR.

10. ABDE

Anti-Kell antibodies seem to affect red cell production rather than causing haemolysis, so amniotic fluid analysis is unreliable. The uniqueness of the antigen-antibody reaction is lost with a change of partner. A critical antibody level is 4 iu/ml. Doppler waveforms may provide guidance in the diagnosis of fetal anaemia but more work is needed. The mirror syndrome is seen in hydrops fetalis; as the baby improves so does the mother's pre-eclamptic toxemia (PET).

11. AC

Information on the detection rates for specific fetal anomalies is extremely difficult to establish from the literature. Spina bifida will probably be detected in 80–90% of cases, but there are variations. Conversely cardiac abnormalities are more likely to be missed. Markers for trisomies may help to detect about 30–40%. Bowel atresia does not usually present till beyond 20 weeks. The lips are not always seen or looked for so clefting may well be missed.

12. AD

Low-dose aspirin (60–75 mg per day) has been utilized in pregnancy in the prophylaxis of pre-eclampsia, the management of primary antiphospholipid syndrome and thromboprophylaxis. Aspirin irreversibly acetylates the cyclo-oxygenase enzyme in platelets and is thought to have its primary action within the presystemic circulation after absorption from the small bowel. Large randomized placebo-controlled double-blind trials have investigated the role of prophylactic low-dose aspirin in the prevention of pre-eclampsia.. The largest of these, Collaborative Low Dose Aspirin Study in Pregnancy (CLASP), showed that those taking aspirin had only a 12% reduction in pre-eclampsia. This was not significant. There was, however, a small but significant reduction in preterm labour. Subgroup analysis of the CLASP trial indicated that a cohort of women with a past history of early-onset pre-eclampsia, essential hypertension (requiring treatment) and renal disease did benefit, in that it prevented early-onset pre-eclampsia.

In the meta-analysis of all prospective randomized double-blind placebo-controlled trials there was no excess of epidural complications, in particular epidural haematomas in patients taking low-dose aspirin. Meta-analysis of all trials in which antiplatelet agents were used in pregnancy suggested that these agents reduce the incidence of deep vein thrombosis and pulmonary embolism by up to 70%.

13. ACD

In appropriately grown fetuses the plasma triglyceride concentration decreases in an exponential way with gestation. In hypoxaemic small for gestational age fetuses, the plasma triglyceride concentrations are increased for a given gestation. Also the blood glucose and plasma insulin levels are decreased and the total non-esterified fatty acid and glycerol levels are not changed. In pregnancies complicated by fetal hypoxaemia and growth retardation there is disturbance in both maternal and fetal plasma amino acid profiles. During hypoxaemia, the fetal plasma concentrations of essential amino acids decrease. However, some non-essential gluconeogenic amino acids and the glycine to valine ratio are increased. For a given gestation, small for gestational age fetuses have raised plasma cortisol levels. Presumably, in a serological sense this is in an effort to combat accompanying hypoglycaemia.

14. ACD

Pregnancy has a major effect on the coagulation and fibrinolytic system. Platelets play an important role in maintaining the integrity of the vascular tree especially at a microscopic level, where they interact with the vascular endothelium. In simple terms the nucleated vascular endothelial cells are a potent source of prostacyclin, which has antiaggregation and secretory activity. Platelets, which are fragments from megakaryocytes, are anuclear cells with a circulating life of approximately 11 days. Activation of platelets may be stimulated by factors such as adenosine diphosphate, adenosine triphosphate, serotonin and other agents such as angiotensin II. Platelets themselves produce a proaggregatory eicosanoid, thromboxane A_2. This tends to enhance any aggregatory effect of the platelets.

Plasma fibrinogen concentrations rise during pregnancy by approximately 50% and, considering the significant increase in plasma volume in pregnancy, this means that there is considerable fibrinogen synthesis. Thrombin activity has a tendency to increase during pregnancy. One of the indicators of this is the increase in Factor VIII antigen:activity ratio. Factor VIII is activated by thrombin and, by doing so, loses its coagulant activity. However, Factor VIII has a continuing antigenic potential so that the increase in antigen relative to coagulation activity is a sign of thrombin activation.

15. CD

The vacuum extractor has been used since its introduction into obstetrics by Malmstrom in 1954. The indications for delivery with vacuum extractor are virtually the same as those used for forceps in the second stage. Contraindications to vacuum extraction include cephalopelvic disproportion; face, brow and breech presentation; and delivery of a premature infant (less than 34 weeks' gestation). A meta-analysis of prospective controlled trials of the use of vacuum extractor versus forceps delivery has noted that failure to deliver with the chosen instrument is more likely to occur in the vacuum extractor group. However, significant maternal trauma (third- and fourth-degree perineal tears and extensive vaginal laceration) and postpartum pain are more common with forceps deliveries. Scalp injury (exclusively cephalohaematomas) and retinal haemorrhages are more commonly associated with use of the vacuum extractor. Two major advantages of using the vacuum extractor are the ease with which it can be applied and the need for less analgesia at delivery. This is particularly true of the new Silastic cups. However, expertise in the use of the instrument is paramount. As with the forceps, the operator should be sure of the position of the fetal head, and no more than one-fifth of the head should be palpable abdominally. Practically speaking, one should first determine whether the patient is suitable for a safe instrumental vaginal delivery, and then decide which instrument is most appropriate.

16. ABDE

Abruptio placentae is caused by separation of the normally implanted placenta before the birth of the fetus. The pathophysiology is initiated most commonly by bleeding into the decidua basalis. The most common source of this bleeding is the small arterial vessels in the basal layer of the decidua.

The reported incidence is variable around the world but the most widely published series based on population studies gives an incidence of between 0.49 and 1.29%. However, abruption severe enough to kill the fetus is less common, being found in 1 in 420 deliveries.

There is anecdotal evidence that abruptio placentae is more common in women that use cocaine recreationally. The alleged reasons for this association may relate to the vasoactive properties of cocaine. In an American series, approximately 5% of women with documented cocaine abuse had abruption as a complication of their pregnancy. Women who have had a previous abruption are at risk of another in a subsequent pregnancy and the recurrence rate has been reported at between 5 and 16%, as much as 30 times the incidence in the general population. After two consecutive abruptions the risk rises to 25%.

17. ACD

ATP is the most common autoimmune bleeding disorder encountered in pregnancy. As with so many autoimmune phenomena, this is so because of a female preponderance of three to one. It is characterized by the production of IgG antibodies which act directly on maternal and fetal platelets. The major site of production in the mother is the spleen. The IgG antibody binds the platelets and renders them more susceptible to sequestration within the reticuloendothelial system. The platelet-associated IgG level correlates directly with the severity of thrombocytopenia in the mother but not in the fetus.

Most women with ATP have a history of easy bruising, petechial haemorrhages and sometimes frank bleeding. The diagnosis is based on four findings: (1) maternal platelet count of less than $100{,}000/mm^3$ with megathrombocytes on peripheral smear; (2) bone marrow examination indicates normal or increased megakaryocyte numbers; (3) no history of drug exposure; and (4) the absence of splenomegaly.

The goal of treatment is to minimize the risk of haemorrhage to the mother and the fetus. The mainstay of therapy is glucocorticoid drugs, the most common of which is prednisolone. This is usually given in divided doses at a dose of 1–2 mg per kg per day. Splenectomy removes the main site of destruction of damaged platelets but carries a large morbidity in pregnancy. However, there are recorded cases of this being combined with caesarean section at term. Intravenous immunoglobulin (400 mg per kg per day for 5 days) has been associated with an increased platelet count.

The risk of fetal thrombocytopenia and bleeding is probably lower than has been previously thought and morbidity is very uncommon in this group. Some workers, particularly in the United States, have advocated percutaneous umbilical cord sampling before delivery to determine platelet count. However, the majority of fetal medicine specialists in the UK would probably not consider this necessary.

18. ABC

Abdominal wound infection following caesarean section is a common occurrence, complicating care in approximately 5% of all women. Prospective studies have suggested an increased incidence in wound infection if the membranes have been ruptured for longer than 6 hours before delivery and is more common in so called 'dirty wounds' if vaginal exogenous contamination has occurred. The most prevalent bacteria in the lower genital tract include the facultative (aerobic) organisms such as Lactobacillaceae, non-haemolytic streptococci, group B β-haemolytic streptococci, *Staphylococcus epidermidis*, *Escherichia coli* and anaerobic bacteria (such as peptococcus, peptostreptococcus and *Bacteroides fragilis*). There is prospective evidence that systemic antibiotics at the time of caesarean section reduce the morbidity from wound infection. However, antibiotic peritoneal lavage with caesarean section appears to be somewhat less effective than systemic antibiotics for the prevention of wound infection (antibiotic peritoneal irrigation versus systemic antibiotics for caesarean section).

Necrotizing fasciitis is an uncommon but serious wound infection. It usually occurs approximately 6–8 days after operation. If response to broad-spectrum antibiotic therapy aimed at mixed aerobic and anaerobic bacteria does not lead to resolution of symptoms, a diagnosis of necrotizing fasciitis should be considered. The necessity for early recognition and extensive surgical debridement as well as specific antibiotic therapy is well documented.

19. ABC

CMV is a DNA virus of the herpes group. Epidemiological data indicate that at least 50% of females in the UK and Europe are susceptible to CMV infection by the time they reach reproductive age. The highest rate of seroconversion occurs between the ages of 13 and 35 years. Past exposure to CMV relates to low socioeconomic status, multiparity, older age, first pregnancy at under 15 years of age, and total number of sexual partners.

Congenital CMV infection is generally the result of transplacental transmission which causes in-utero infection. Between 0.5 and 2.5% of the neonatal population are infected by vertical transmission from mother to fetus. Up to 50% of neonates whose mothers have congenital CMV infection at the time of birth will acquire the virus. The prognosis is poor for babies who have clinically apparent disease at birth. Infection of the central nervous system usually results in severe mental retardation.

The general consensus holds that routine antepartum screening for CMV infection is not indicated. However, if in-utero CMV infection is suspected, anti-CMV IgM in fetal blood may be diagnostic, and more recent studies have demonstrated that the detection of the virus in amniotic fluid is highly sensitive. It is thus recommended that amniotic fluid culture for CMV should be obtained in those pregnant women who have documented primary CMV infection or ultrasound findings making the physician suspicious of in-utero infection.

No effective treatment for maternal CMV infection is approved and clinically available. However, attempts have been made to use antiviral drugs such as arabinoside and cytosine arabinoside.

20. ACE

Sacral coccygeal teratoma (SCT) is the most common tumour of the newborn with an estimated incidence of 1 in 35,000 live births. Before routine ultrasonography was available, the majority of cases remained asymptomatic in utero and were diagnosed after birth. However, with the advent of routine mid-trimester scans, the diagnosis has become more frequently made prenatally. The main complication in utero is the occurrence of hydrops due to high output cardiac failure in the fetus secondary to a vascular steal. In a series from the United States, 45% of fetuses with these prenatally diagnosed anomalies died in utero or at birth. Presentation after 30 weeks' gestation is a relatively good prognostic sign.

The tumour mass may be associated with polyhydramnios and in some circumstances the maternal 'mirror syndrome' (a situation where the mother mirrors the fetal hydropic state with hypertension, oedema and renal dysfunction) may occur. Problems with delivery of the fetus secondary to tumour bulk may be anticipated.

21. CDE

In diamniotic-monochorionic placentation the placental masses and chorion are fused, and their dividing membrane consists of two translucent amnions only. When they are separated from each other, the single chorion on the placental surface is apparent. In the past it has been thought that these placentas contain various types of interfetal vascular communications. However, recent studies have indicated that this is not so. However, such twin placentation is associated with twin–twin transfusion syndrome, polyhydramnios–oligohydramnios sequence and an overall perinatal mortality rate of 25%.

22. ABD

HIV is one of five human retroviruses known and is a single-stranded RNA envelope virus. The incidence of new infection seems to be increasing rapidly among women and comprise of 11% of the total number of women infected in the United States and in Britain. More than 80% of cases of paediatric AIDS are secondary to vertical transmission of HIV from mother to fetus, although prenatal transmission transplacentally is 14–50%. Recent studies from this country have indicated that symptomatic seropositive women, compared with sero-negative controls have no difference in pregnancy outcome except for an increased risk of spontaneous miscarriage. However, in this study, the incidence of prematurity and low birthweight babies in both groups of intravenous drug users was about twice that recorded for the general population. These data are concordant with those from other international studies. At present, a significant influence of pregnancy on the course of HIV disease has not been documented. However, a prospective long-term study is underway investigating the impact of pregnancy on the disease, so that any adverse factors can be clearly delineated. It is important that HIV-infected women adhere rigorously to the standards of care for all HIV-infected individuals. These women should receive Pneumovax, influenza and hepatitis vaccines, and should be screened for tuberculosis and sexually transmitted diseases. The immune status should be monitored by CD4 count, which should be performed every trimester. If the count drops under 500 cells/ mm^3, consideration should be given to the use of azidothymidine (AZT) to delay the onset of clinical illness. However, prospective phase 2 trials have not yet been mounted for this therapy. If the count were to drop lower than this, *Pneumocystis carnipneumona* prophylaxis should be instituted.

23. AD

In the UK anti-D maternal red cell alloimmunization is still the most common morbid cause of haemolytic disease of the newborn. However, the incidence has decreased markedly since the introduction of immune globulin. Red cell destruction by anti-D (either IgM or IgG) is by a non-complement-mediated mechanism. The anti-D attaches to the erythrocyte membrane and chemotaxis is increased. The red cells adhere to macrophages, so causing red cell destruction.

The majority of alloimmunized women are monitored by regular determination of antibody titres, ultrasonography and possibly amniotic fluid monitoring at OD450. However, rapid in utero intravascular transfusion has revolutionized the management of the most severely affected fetuses. Transfusion in many centres is not started until at least 20 weeks' gestation. Therefore, several intermediate modalities have been used to try to suppress rhesus alloimmunization. Both plasma exchange and high-dose immunoglobulin therapy have been utilized and shown to reduce the circulating maternal IgG concentration. There is little objective evidence that this improves perinatal survival.

Studies from Canada have indicated that one prophylactic dose of rhesus immunoglobulin (300 μg) is beneficial if given to rhesus-negative unimmunized pregnant women at 28 weeks' gestation. This is repeated if delivery has not occurred within 12.5 weeks after this injection.

24. ACE

Babies who are small at birth and during infancy are known to be at increased risk of cardiovascular disease during adulthood, in particular coronary heart disease, hypertension and non-insulin-dependent diabetes. These data have been prospectively noted from cohort studies in central England. People that were small at birth have raised blood pressure and raised serum cholesterol levels as adults. Abdominal circumference is also indirectly correlated with serum cholesterol and total low density lipoprotein concentrations. Placental weight is also correlated with adult disease, independently with birthweight. Babies with a placenta that is disproportionally large in relation to their weight are at increased risk from cardiovascular disease, high blood pressure and impaired glucose tolerance. In adapting to undernutrition, the fetus restricts its growth in order to survive, but this occurs at the expense of longevity.

25. BDE

The antenatal recognition of IUGR is a primary aim of obstetric care. However, detection of this potentially catastrophic problem in utero may have no effect on perinatal mortality and morbidity. Abdominal circumference and estimated fetal weight are better predictors of small for gestational age babies at birth than biparietal diameter, head circumference: abdominal circumference ratio and femur length:abdominal circumference ratio. In high-risk women, an abdominal circumference of less than the 10th centile predicts at least 85% of small for gestational age fetuses.

Umbilical artery and uteroplacental Doppler waveforms are inferior to abdominal circumference and estimated fetal weight in the prediction of small for gestational babies at birth. In high-risk populations, the sensitivity for umbilical artery systolic:diastolic ratio greater than 3 is 53%. Limited data on fetal Doppler waveforms from the aorta and middle cerebral circulation suggest that these may be more predictive. The results of five randomized controlled trials of ultrasonography in late pregnancy, whether low or high risk, have indicated that isolated measurements of fetal size by ultrasonography do not improve fetal outcome in terms of morbidity and mortality.

26. E

Fluid retention can be manifested as a rapid gain in weight before demonstrable oedema. However, rapid weight gain can occur in pregnancy without pre-eclampsia. Characteristically, the oedema of pre-eclampsia is non-dependent, i.e. it is seen in the hands and face. This is considered to be related to sodium retention, whereas dependent oedema is a function of hydrostatic mechanisms. However, oedema of the hands and face occurs in 10–15% of women whose blood pressure remains normal throughout pregnancy. In severe pre-eclampsia, significant hypoalbuminuria may further exacerbate the sodium retention and massive oedema can result.

Evidence supports serum uric acid concentration as a useful confirmatory marker for pre-eclampsia. However, its discriminatory value as a predictor of pre-eclampsia remains to be proved.

Chronic hypertension is present in approximately 1–5% of pregnancies.

The rationale for the use of antihypertensive therapy in mild pre-eclampsia is not to lower blood pressure, but to improve perinatal outcome by prolonging pregnancy safely in patients who are distant from term. However, there is little evidence to suggest that antihypertensive therapy is of use in the management of mild pre-eclampsia remote from term. Comparative trials between hydralazine, nifedipine and labetalol have not shown any of these agents to be superior in the acute management of severe hypertension in pregnancy.

27. AB

The results of the CLASP trial did not support the widespread routine prophylactic or therapeutic use of antiplatelet therapy in pregnancy among all women judged to be at risk of pre-eclampsia or IUGR. The only women in whom the use of low-dose aspirin might be justified are those at especially high risk of early-onset pre-eclampsia (i.e. before 32 weeks' gestation). As it is not possible to identify such women prospectively, those with a previous history of early-onset pre-eclampsia might be considered to be susceptible.

The association of pre-eclampsia with haemolysis, raised levels of liver enzymes and low platelet count has long been recognized. This triad of parameters was labelled with the acronym of HELLP. The incidence of HELLP in women with pre-eclampsia is reported to vary between 4 and 12%.

Patients with HELLP syndrome have increased maternal morbidity and mortality rate and the reported perinatal mortality rate ranges from approximately 8% to 37%.

The risk of chronic hypertension after pregnancy complicated with pregnancy-induced hypertension or pre-eclampsia is reported to be considerably increased. The presence of hypertension at follow-up is closely related to residual renal disorder.

28. D

Controversy exists concerning the place of amniocentesis in the management of rhesus disease. First described in the 1960s, many data exist now concerning its utility. Liley's charts started only at 27 weeks but the Whitfield Action line commenced at 20 weeks, and more recently data exist from 16 weeks. An anti-D concentration of 4 iu/ml is usually taken as the threshold for amniocentesis. The key to the use of amniotic fluid is that at least two points on the chart are required to enable extrapolation. One advantage of the method is that it gives an indication of the progress of the haemolytic process. Even a falling level, however, does not exclude an affected baby and a rise in antibody concentration indicates the need for a further amniocentesis. A rising delta OD does not necessarily indicate delivery. Amniotic fluid analysis does not appear to be of value in determining anti-Kell antibodies, whose mode of action seems different from that of anti-D.

29. AD

Past obstetric history is at best only a guide to the severity of rhesus disease. The antigen-antibody interaction that produces the haemolysis is unique so, if the partnership is new, past history ceases to be of any value. A single amniotic fluid result is of little value unless it is very high, and an antibody level of 10 iu/ml does not indicate severity *per se*. Ultrasonography can be used to indicate the extent of fetal involvement from subtle evidence of fluid in abdominal and pericardial cavities and also changes in Doppler waveform patterns. Using ultrasonography in this way may delay the use of invasive tests but the examination requires skill and equipment of good quality. By the time gross ascites appears the fetus is already sick and will usually have a haemoglobin level of around 3.0 g/dl. Direct evidence of fetal anaemia can be obtained from cordocentesis but this should be the preserve of referral centres.

30. ABCDE

Anaerobic bacteria and *Ureaplasma urealyticum* have been shown to produce large amounts of phospholipase A_2 which is capable of initiating prostaglandin synthesis by cleaving arachidonic acid from the phospholipid components of fetal membranes. *Neisseria gonorrhoeae* and *Chlamydia trachomatis* infections have been associated with preterm labour and delivery but a causal mechanism has yet to be proven.

31. BCE

Gardnerella vaginalis and *Ureaplasma urealyticum* are correlated with bacterial vaginosis. Bacterial vaginosis is associated with a high vaginal pH and preterm labour and delivery.

32. C

Prospective randomized trials have shown that induction at 41 weeks and beyond decreases caesarean section rates. Vaginal instrumental delivery rates are increased by a policy of induction at 40 weeks but unaltered at 41+ weeks. The incidence of meconium-stained liquor is reduced but this does not affect the incidence of meconium aspiration. Neonatal seizures are unaffected by these induction policies.

33. AB

Prophylactic forceps were once considered advantageous for delivery of the premature fetus because they were thought to act as a protective 'cage', relieving pressure on the head from the pelvic floor. Clinical studies have shown this not to be the case. Elective episiotomy with a spontaneous delivery is now considered the best management. Neonatal cephalhaematoma is associated with vacuum delivery and facial palsy is a recognized complication of forceps delivery, but not in the mother.

34. A

Randomized clinical trials show a shorter labour from early amniotomy but this amounts to little more than an hour and has no effect on intervention (caesarean or operative vaginal delivery), no reduction in the use of oxytocin, no change in analgesia requirement, and no improvement in neonatal outcome.

35. E

Routine early amniotomy speeds up progress in labour but does not affect intervention or outcome. Oxytocin acceleration to return slow progress to normal without regard to aetiology confers no benefits and increases the need for analgesia. Epidural analgesia has long been the subject of debate regarding increased need for operative intervention. Randomized trials tend to confirm increased need for operative intervention in both first and second stages of labour. Continuous electronic fetal monitoring in low-risk cases does not improve neonatal outcome and is associated with 'false positives', which increase caesarean section rates, particularly when not backed up with fetal blood sampling.

36. BCE

Amnio-infusion improves neonatal blood gases and Apgar scores but this does not lead to improvement in mortality. There does not appear to be an increased incidence of maternal infection.

37. CD

About 60% of breeches can be turned successfully at 37 weeks. At this gestational age, less than 1% will revert to a breech presentation and a further 10% will require caesarean section. Therefore, given today's low threshold for caesarean section, the probability of caesarean delivery is likely to be halved. Uterine rupture is a well recognized risk, albeit very rare. Rhesus-negative women should receive anti-D immunoglobulins and have a Kleihauer test to quantify any fetomaternal haemorrhage.

Version should not be performed under sedation or anaesthesia (because maternal discomfort limits the force used) and facilities for caesarean section should be readily available in case of complications such as persistent bradycardia or rupture of membranes with cord prolapse.

38. AE

The risk of scar rupture or dehiscence is about 0.8%. The earliest warning is fetal heart rate abnormalities.

Erect lateral pelvimetry, in today's population, provides little prognostic information and may result in overintervention, depending on cut-off limits. This applies even to cases where caesarean delivery was performed for 'failure to progress'.

Intrauterine pressure monitoring carries no safeguards in itself and the information it provides has to be interpreted very carefully lest it be misleading. Repetition frequency and timing of duration of contractions by an experienced midwife should give a good, clinically useful, index of uterine activity in all but the most obese of patients.

39. ABCDE

Any subsequent labour after a lower segment caesarean section should be conducted in a well-equipped maternity hospital with ready access to caesarean section. The labouring woman should be attended by an experienced midwife or doctor and the fetal heart rate should be monitored continuously.

40. C

The routine vaginal examination at the 6-week postnatal visit has no medical basis and is unlikely to reveal findings that will affect the management of an a symptomatic woman. There is also a high incidence (up to 35%) of false-positive (inflammatory) cervical smears, and whenever possible smears should be collected after 12 weeks postnatally. As over 50% of women would have resumed ovulation and sexual intercourse by 6 weeks, the ideal time for starting contraception is at 3 weeks postnatally.

Despite the common misconception that the majority of childbirth-related health problems resolve by 6 weeks postnatally, it has been recently shown that almost 50% of postnatal women develop at least one health problem lasting more than 6 weeks; most of these problems start within 1 week of delivery and 70% last for over 1 year. These include backache, migraine, urinary frequency and incontinence, depression and anxiety.

41. ABCDE

The finding of breech presentation at term should be investigated by a detailed ultrasonographic scan as it is associated with fetal anomalies. This should be done even if the woman has had a normal mid-trimester scan; anomalies could have developed later on and an error in the first scan is a possibility. Breech presentation is also associated with placenta praevia, which is another reason for the scan. Having said that, the commonest site of placentation in the term breech is the cornual region.

There is increased perinatal mortality and morbidity in babies presenting with the breech at term, irrespective of the mode of delivery.

Congenital uterine abnormalities (in the mother) are associated with breech presentation. Women with these abnormalities tend to have breech presentation in successive pregnancies.

42. ABCE

Atrial fibrillation is pathological and should always be investigated. Rotation of the heart due to elevation of the diaphragm raises the apex beat from the 5th to the 4th intercostal space. Flow murmurs are common owing to increased circulation of blood through the heart and the blood becomes less viscous, therefore becoming more turbulent in its flow. Ectopic beats are a not uncommon finding and may be described as palpitations.

43. ACD

Pregnancy is a hypercoagulable state, with an increase in the risk of venous thromboembolism from about 5 in 100,000 non-pregnant women per year to 60 in 100,000 during pregnancy.

High progesterone levels do not increase the risk of thromboembolism. Due to physiological haemodilution in pregnancy there is a fall in blood viscosity which should, under normal circumstances, decrease the propensity to thromboembolism.

44. ABE

Glomerular filtration rises by up to 60% early in the first trimester. Glucose filtration rises, presenting the tubule with a larger load, which can lead to glycosuria. Similarly, other nutrients such as amino acids and folic acid can be lost from the blood. In the urine they constitute a good culture medium for infection. Urea and creatinine are filtered by the kidney and their concentrations fall as a result of increased glomerular filtration.

45. ABCE

The oxygen-carrying capacity of the blood slightly exceeds the demand of the conceptus (15–20%), resulting in venous blood being slightly more saturated with oxygen than in the non-pregnant state.

Cardiac output exceeds the demand for oxygenated blood and probably has more to do with getting rid of excretory products such as carbon dioxide, urea and heat.

The fall in haemoglobin concentration in normal pregnancy is physiological, whereas anaemia is, by definition, pathological. The old term 'normal anaemia of pregnancy' was discarded long ago.

Mild dyspnoea is common owing to hyperventilation resulting from the stimulatory effect of raised progesterone levels on the respiratory centre.

46. ACDE

Some 15–50% of cases of uterine inversion occur after the third stage and 90% are associated with postpartum haemorrhage. Urinary retention is common and should be resolved by catheterization before repositioning; and once the uterus has been returned to its correct position, it should be explored for trauma.

47. ACD

Amniotic fluid embolism can occur before amniotomy. Presumably some defect in the membranes must occur to permit ingress of the liquor to the circulation but it may not be clinically detectable. The condition is more common in women of high parity. It is a difficult diagnosis to make with certainty until post-mortem examination of the lungs. It is said to carry a 50% mortality rate, but this may reflect underdiagnosis of non-fatal cases.

48. D

Both clinical and erect lateral radiographic pelvimetry rarely detect pelvic pathology and there is some evidence to suggest that radiographic pelvimetry may cause unnecessary intervention. Cervimetry is an aid to the management of labour. Retrospective analysis may be interesting but it rarely identifies specific pathology. The chances of the woman delivering vaginally next time are of the order of 60%.

49. A

Symptomless bacteriuria ($>10^5$ organisms per ml urine) is present in 3–8% of pregnant women. If untreated, 15–45% of these women will develop acute cystitis or pyelonephritis. Screening for asymptomatic bacteriuria during pregnancy is therefore standard practice in developed countries. Culture and colony count of a single voided midstream specimen is the best currently available form of screening for bacteriuria.

Recognition and treatment of asymptomatic bacteriuria in pregnancy will result in a substantially reduced risk of acute pyelonephritis. It also appears to reduce the incidence of preterm delivery and low birthweight, although this relationship is somewhat more tenuous. The available evidence suggests that sulphonamides, nitrofurantoin, ampicillin and the first-generation cephalosporins are equally effective in the treatment. Tetracyclines are contraindicated during pregnancy as they interfere with the development of bones in the fetus and predispose to acute fatty liver in the mother.

50. BC

Dexon (polyglycolic acid) is a high molecular weight linear polymer of hydroxyacetic (glycolic) acid. One-third of its breaking strength is lost at 7 days; complete absorption occurs in 90–120 days. The Cochrane Obstetric database identified 14 controlled trials of perineal suturing following vaginal delivery. The meta-analysis of these trials concluded that Dexon and Vicryl are superior to catgut because they produce significantly less pain, less need for analgesia and less late dyspareunia. Compared with catgut, polyglycolic acid sutures were associated with about a 40% reduction in short-term pain and need for analgesia.

51. CE

The use of forceps to assist the delivery of the after-coming head in breech presentation is well recognized. Forceps should not be applied to the mentoposterior presentation because safe vaginal delivery is impossible as such. The forceps used to assist delivery of the fetal head in caesarean section is often wrongly assumed to be Wrigley's forceps. Wrigley's forceps has both pelvic and cephalic curves, whereas the forceps used in caesarean section is a straight, short shanked forceps; it has no pelvic curve, hence the two blades look exactly the same.

Early in the twentieth century, Joseph DeLee proposed the

use of prophylactic forceps to protect the fetal skull and its contents from the trauma of delivery. Although the concept became quite popular, particularly in relation to delivery of the preterm infant, conclusive scientific proof of the validity of this idea has never been established. Indeed, in an infant weighing less than 1500 g, routine forceps delivery (in cases where there is no specific indication) offers no advantage and may in fact be deleterious owing to increased incidence of intracranial bleeding. Spontaneous delivery with a generous episiotomy and manual control appears preferable.

52. CD

Neither the vacuum extractor nor the obstetric forceps should be applied until the presentation and position are identified; a policy of 'pull and see' with the vacuum extractor in cases where the position is not identified is improper. The vacuum extractor has been shown to be associated with significantly less maternal trauma than forceps, and it has been suggested that it should be the first choice for instrumental vaginal delivery.

53. ACDE

The 'decision to delivery' interval is similar for forceps and vacuum extractor, although the range is greater for forceps. This is at least in part due to the time required to institute the more complex forms of analgesia used for forceps delivery.

The widely held belief that vacuum extraction is too slow to be useful when rapid delivery is required for fetal distress can be laid firmly to rest.

Vacuum extraction is more likely to cause cephalhaematoma than forceps, but forceps are more likely to cause other kinds of scalp and fetal injuries.

54. AC

During the period 1985–1990 the estimated fatality rate per 1000 caesarean sections in the UK was 0.33 (i.e. 3.3 per 10,000 caesarean deliveries).

In one prospective study a significant negative correlation between perceived delivery difficulty and incision size was reported. An abdominal incision size of 15 cm or more was associated with significantly less difficulty in caesarean delivery. Pfannenstiel incision of less than 13 cm in diameter was associated with a perceived difficulty of fetal delivery.

The available information from controlled trials suggests that manual removal of the placenta increases maternal blood loss. Elective manual removal of placenta during caesarean section should be avoided, particularly in Rhesus-negative women and others in whom transplacental bleeding might increase the risk of isosensitization.

The available evidence suggests that the results of one-layer and two-layer uterine closure are similar. A policy of uterine exteriorization before repair results in somewhat lower blood loss than repairing the uterus while in the pelvis.

55. AC

The best mode of delivery for the preterm breech (26–32 weeks' gestation) remains uncertain and will have to await performance of a properly conducted trial, which in the light of current experience seems unlikely ever to be performed. In the absence of such evidence, the decision about the mode of delivery should be reached after close consultation with the labouring woman and her partner.

Closure of visceral or parietal peritoneum is not necessary. When left undisturbed peritoneal defects demonstrate mesothelial integrity within 48 hours and indistinguishable healing with no scar by 5 days.

Caesarean section, even under ideal conditions, is still a major operation and has its associated mortality and morbidity.

56. CE

The outcome of cardiopulmonary resuscitation in the pregnant patient is less successful with a longer time to restore spontaneous circulation and an increased mortality rate. The principal reason for this is the hazard presented by aortocaval compression. The patient therefore needs to be positioned so that the uterus is wedged and yet such that effective thoracic compression is still achievable. Caesarean section may be indicated for maternal survival by removing the source of caval compression, as well as for potential fetal survival. High doses of bupivacaine are associated with cardiac arrest from which successful resuscitation is particularly difficult. Endotracheal intubation is indicated to prevent gastric aspiration as well as a means of providing artificial ventilation.

57. All the answers are false

Convulsions are less likely to occur because of the lower dose of local anaesthetic required for spinal block. The duration of spinal block is significantly shorter and, because it is not usually possible to insert an intrathecal catheter, an unusually difficult caesarean section should be anticipated, so that an epidural catheter can be inserted before the operation commences. The degree of sympathetic block is the same by whichever route the local anaesthetic is given, although the speed of onset of block of all modalities is quicker with spinal administration. With the newer type of spinal needles the likelihood of postdural puncture headache is broadly similar whether an epidural or a spinal is used, given the incidence of inadvertent dural tap from an epidural, although the actual incidence will vary from unit to unit. The onset of action of local anaesthesia is quicker by the spinal route.

58. D

Although the headache can present soon after the tap, it can also present up to 2–3 days later. A postdural puncture headache is relieved by recumbency and hence is usually better early in the morning, although this does depend on how much the mother has been up attending to her baby during the night! Paracetamol is not usually effective. Firm abdominal pressure (Gutsche test) relieves the headache almost immediately and is a useful diagnostic test. Preventing straining in the second stage of labour by elective forceps or caesarean delivery used to be practised but this merely delayed the onset of headache.

59. ACE

Sensory innervation of the uterus is via visceral afferent fibres which traverse the uterine, cervical and hypogastric plexuses to the 11th and 12th thoracic nerve roots with some overlap to the 10th thoracic and 1st lumbar nerve roots. The dermatome that corresponds to the 10th thoracic nerve root is at the umbilicus. Thus skin testing of an epidural block can reveal whether the block is sufficiently extensive. The pudendal nerves (second to fourth sacral segments) are involved with sensory innervation of the vagina, vulva and perineum, and hence are related to pain in the second stage of labour. Paracervical block can be used to achieve analgesia in the first stage of labour but its major disadvantage is the relatively high frequency of fetal bradycardia.

60. AD

Failed intubation occurs in approximately 1 in 280 obstetric anaesthetics compared with 1 in 2230 general surgical patients. The reasons for this include breast enlargement making laryngoscope insertion difficult, abnormal positioning because of lateral tilt and cricoid pressure application, and in some cases laryngeal and pharyngeal oedema. Antacid prophylaxis is important in the prevention of acid aspiration but it is cricoid pressure that stems back any regurgitated gastric contents. The volatile agents, isoflurane, enflurane and halothane, relax the uterus. This property can be put to good use to aid obstetric access, for example in preterm delivery where the lower segment is unformed, where there is a transverse lie or a breech presentation in labour. However, this uterine relaxation property means that the average blood loss is approximately double that under regional blockade. Preoperative assessment of the patient's medical condition, airway access, allergies, complications of pregnancy, etc. are vital. When speed is of the essence, safety for the mother cannot be compromised but the obstetrician can help the anaesthetist by giving prior warning of potential problems (e.g. at an antenatal visit) and by giving the anaesthetist a concise relevant history when requesting emergency anaesthesia. This is all in the patient's interests.

61. CE

Entonox is a mixture of 50% nitrous oxide in oxygen. If it were mixed with air the mixture would be hypoxic. To be effective the mother needs to breathe it as soon as the contraction starts and before the painful phase of the contraction. Since the withdrawal of methoxyflurane and trichloroethylene, Entonox is now the only approved inhalational method of analgesia. Nitrous oxide is very insoluble and hence it is all exhaled between contractions and there is no accumulation. Entonox is a compressed gas provided the temperature remains above 7°C. At this temperature the nitrous oxide liquefies, resulting in an oxygen-rich gas being emitted initially, followed by a hypoxic nitrous oxide-rich gas. Thus it is important that nitrous oxide cylinders are stored above this critical temperature.

62. ABCDE

By reducing the activity of the enzyme cyclo-oxygenase, non-steroidal anti-inflammatory agents inhibit the synthesis and release of prostaglandins, prostacyclins and thromboxane, which sensitize pain receptors to mechanical stimulation or to other pain mediators. They are a useful adjunct in the management of postoperative pain, reducing the opioid requirement and hence their side-effects. However, they do need to be used with care because they can provoke renal failure; hence they should not be used in pre-eclampsia or after massive haemorrhage. They can also cause gastric erosions or ulceration.

63. AB

Recently published data by the Eclampsia Trial Collaborative Group have shown that magnesium sulphate is more effective than diazepam and phenytoin in preventing recurrence of eclampsia. Magnesium sulphate 40 mg/kg intravenously, before induction of anaesthesia, has been shown to be effective in obtunding the pressor response to intubation in pre-eclamptics. It enhances the effect of muscle relaxants, particularly non-depolarizing muscle relaxants. There is doubt as to its effect on depolarizing muscle relaxants (i.e. suxamethonium). Although magnesium sulphate produces widespread vasodilatation, it rarely produces hypotension as there is an increase in cardiac output to combat this. It is reversed by calcium, not potassium, chloride.

64. BDE

Anaemia is better tolerated than hypovolaemia. Rapid fluid infusion takes priority over the choice of fluid. One of the main aims of resuscitation is to restore the circulating blood volume to a CVP approaching the normal value of 0–5 cmH_2O. There should not be a formula for giving clotting factors but these should be administered on the basis of coagulation results. The pregnant woman has an increased circulating volume and can tolerate a loss of up to 1500 ml without any change in blood pressure. When adequate resuscitation has occurred, there is minimal difference between peripheral and core temperatures, and maintaining body temperature by active warming is again a part of the resuscitation process.

65. BCDE

Typically postdural puncture headache is characterized by a postural frontal or occipital headache relieved by lying supine and worsened on assuming the upright position. The incidence of postdural puncture headache is reduced by using pencil point needles for subarachnoid anaesthesia. Caffeine relieves the headache by causing vasoconstriction. The headache is a low-pressure cerebrospinal fluid headache due to leakage, which in turn gives rise to vasodilatation. The headache is relieved by epidural blood patching in 86% of cases.

66. BD

Ambulatory epidurals are a combined spinal epidural in which a combination of bupivacaine and fentanyl are used to produce rapid onset of analgesia without motor blockade. Lack of motor loss or ability to mobilize in labour has been shown to enhance maternal satisfaction. There has not yet been any evidence to show that there is a decreased incidence of either caesarean section or forceps delivery as a result of increased mobility.

67. A

Epidurals diminish the cardiovascular response to pain and prevent tachycardia and hypertensive swings during contractions and are, therefore, indicated with previous MI. Epidurals can also be detrimental in certain cardiac condition as sympathetic blockade and hypotension with decreased venous return and reduced cardiac output can occur. Systemic absorption of local anaesthetic can also cause cardiac depression and decreased cardiac output. A high block can give rise to a bradycardia. Basically epidurals are of benefit where it is desirable to produce peripheral vasodilatation and decrease afterload. They are therefore contraindicated in any situation where hypotension cannot be compensated for because of a fixed output as in aortic stenosis or HOCM, or where there would be a reversal of shunt as in Eisenmenger's syndrome. In pulmonary hypertension right ventricular failure can occur with preloading.

68. C

It is not advisable to insert an epidural at the site of the spina bifida occulta as there is an increased likelihood of dural puncture, but the lesion *per se* is not a contraindication to an epidural. Multiple sclerosis is a disease of relapses and remissions, and frequently relapses during the puerperium. There is no scientific evidence that an epidural influences its course, and an epidural could be beneficial if the mother has muscular weakness and fatigues easily. If inadvertent dural puncture occurs, coning may result in the presence of raised intracranial pressure, and for this reason epidural anaesthesia is contraindicated.

In myasthenia gravis the patient will fatigue easily and also be on oral medication to enhance muscle power. Epidural anaesthesia will allow oral mediation to be continued, conserve muscular energy and avoid general anaesthesia which could result in postoperative ventilation being required.

69. ABCE

Normally suxamethonium is short lived: 3–5 minutes in duration. However, if there is an abnormal or absent enzyme, its duration of action can be as long as 24 hours and the mother will require ventilation for that period of time. General anaesthesia should thus be avoided in those who are known to be suxamethonium sensitive. An episode of MH can be triggered by general anaesthesia, particularly the agents used for rapid sequence induction and maintenance of anaesthesia in obstetrics. If a member of a family is suxamethonium sensitive or suffers an episode of MH, first-degree relatives must be investigated. Cricoid pressure involves pressing the cricoid ring perpendicularly against the sixth cervical vertebra, thus obliterating the upper end of the oesophagus. Pressure on the thyroid cartilage can lead to distortion of the larynx and difficulty in intubation. Morbidity and mortality from aspiration of stomach content are dependent on both the acidity and the volume of the contents, acidity being the main determining factor. The morbidity rate is 100% if the pH is 1.5 or less.

70. AE

As is to be expected, adding an inhalational agent to a combination of oxygen and nitrous oxide reduces the risk of maternal awareness and, by reducing the stress response, increases or maintains uteroplacental flow. Low concentrations do not interfere with uterine contractility and thus do not give rise to increased blood loss at caesarean section. This dose is insufficient to obtund maternal awareness during caesarean section if 100% oxygen is used and thus an increased percentage is necessary if 100% oxygen is to be used for fetal benefit.

71. E

Pethidine is loosely bound to α_1-glycoprotein, which has a lower concentration in the fetus than in the mother. Norpethidine has a longer half-life than pethidine (18 hours compared with 3–4 hours).

Naloxone will reverse the effects of pethidine only if given in a relatively large dose: 0.2 mg intramuscularly.

Fentanyl is used in obstetrics because of its lack of respiratory depression and the fact that respiratory depression occurs early, if at all. It is absorbed intravenously and thus has a similar effect on gastric emptying as systemic opiates.

72. ABCE

In the presence of pulmonary oedema, Swan-Ganz catheterization and measurement of pulmonary capillary wedge pressure (PCWP) is an accurate way of assessing left ventricular function and thus instituting appropriate treatment such as fluid restriction, diuretics or inotropes.

Despite the fact that there may be no direct correlation between CVP and PCWP, pulmonary oedema occurs only if the CVP is above 6 mmHg. As protein leaks out of the capillaries in pre-eclampsia, infusions of crystalloid have produced low oncotic pressure pulmonary oedema. One of the signs of impending pulmonary oedema may be a decrease in oxygen saturation. The use of diuretics in the presence of volume depletion associated with pre-eclampsia has led to patient 'collapse'.

73. BDE

Pulmonary thromboembolism (PTE) is a major cause of maternal mortality and in up to 70% of cases there are no previous signs of deep venous thrombosis (DVT). Prevention strategies include the identification of patients with risk factors and the provision of appropriate thromboprophylaxis. These risk factors include: age, high parity, caesarean section (particularly emergency sections in labour), immobilization, dehydration, hypertensive disorders, excessive blood loss, sickle cell anaemia and having a blood group other than O. Patients at particularly high risk are those with thrombophilia, either hereditary (antithrombin III deficiency, protein S deficiency, protein C deficiency and APC resistance) or acquired (such as those with lupus anticoagulants).

74. ADE

Appendicitis has an incidence of about 1 in every 2000 pregnancies, which is similar to that in the non-pregnant population. However, as the diagnosis is more difficult to make during pregnancy, it is associated with a higher mortality rate. This difficulty in diagnosis is due to many factors: usual symptoms such as nausea, vomiting and anorexia are common in pregnancy; the enlarged gravid uterus pushes the appendix outward towards the flank, and hence the pain and tenderness may not be present in the right lower quadrant; some leucocytosis is normal during pregnancy; and finally other conditions (such as placental abruption and pyelonephritis) may be readily confused with appendicitis.

The treatment is always surgical, and the diagnosis is confirmed at surgery in about 70% of cases. Because of the seriousness of the condition, a rate of 30% of normal appendices at laparotomy is thought to be justified.

75. AE

Epilepsy affects 0.5–1% of the population of childbearing age. There is a small increased risk of fetal abnormalities in children of mothers with epilepsy and this risk is further increased if the mother is taking antiepileptic drugs. The number of antiepileptic drugs taken concurrently is important; the risk of fetal abnormalities rises from about double the background risk (2–3% in the general population) in women taking two drugs to a nearly tenfold increase in those taking four drugs. The commonest abnormalities are cleft lip and congenital heart disease. It is therefore advisable that epileptic women of childbearing age should be on the lowest possible dose of a single drug. Sodium valproate is associated with about a 1.5% risk of neural tube defect (NTD) and should be avoided. Carbamazepine is preferable, but it still has about 0.5% risk of NTD. Folic acid supplements should be given and may reduce the risk.

An epileptic mother has a 3–4% chance of having a child who will develop epilepsy before the age of 20 years. Having an epileptic father has the same effect. If there is an epileptic sibling, the risk is 10%, and if both parents are epileptic it is 15–20%. Of course these risk predictions hold true for idiopathic epilepsy; women (and men) with acquired epilepsy (such as after head trauma) impart no increased risk to their children.

Sodium valproate is excreted in breast milk but only in low concentration and does not contraindicate breastfeeding. The concentration received by the breastfed infant is much less than that received by the fetus in utero.

Neither epilepsy nor antiepileptic drugs increase the risk of miscarriage. The increased risk of seizures during or after labour is usually due to failure to take medication, lack of sleep, hyperventilation, or impaired drug absorption.

76. B

Transverse lie of the second twin could be managed by internal podalic version and breech extraction, particularly as the birth canal would have been dilated by delivery of the first twin.

About 60–70% of women undergoing a trial of vaginal delivery after previous caesarean section (including those in whom the indication was cephalopelvic disproportion) will have a successful vaginal delivery.

Mortality due to cord prolapse is the mortality of delay. In the second stage of labour, if safe instrumental delivery is possible, vaginal delivery is the treatment of choice for cord prolapse.

In cases of gastroschisis there is no evidence that caesarean section confers better protection to the fetal gut compared with vaginal delivery. More important is to arrange delivery in a unit with ready access to neonatal surgical care.

77. DE

Acute pancreatitis is rather uncommon during pregnancy (1 in 4000 to 1 in 11,000). Predisposing factors generally include gallstones, familial hyperlipidaemia, hyperparathyroidism and drug ingestion (particularly tetracyclines and thiazide diuretics). Ultrasonographic evidence of gallstones is present in over 50% of cases of pancreatitis in pregnancy, in which they are by far the commonest predisposing factor. The presence of gallstones may make the diagnosis of cholecystitis also probable, but both cases are managed conservatively, with supportive care, pain control, attention to intravenous fluids and electrolyte balance.

78. CD

The BPP score was first described by Frank Manning in Winnipeg, Canada. Originally it consisted of five parameters: four biophysical variables observed on ultrasonography and a non-stress test (cardiotocography), which are each assigned a score of 0 or 2. After the first 30,000 high-risk pregnancies ,it was found that the incidence of abnormal scores based on ultrasonography was about 2% and that dropping the CTG had no deleterious effect on sensitivity or specificity. A score of 8/8 (or 10/10 when CTG is used) is associated with a perinatal mortality rate of 0.7 per 1000. A score of 8/10, where the two points are lost for any parameter apart from the amniotic fluid volume (AFV), is also associated with a perinatal mortality rate of 0.7 per 1000. However, when the 8/10 score is obtained because of abnormally low AFV, the rate is 89 per 1000.

The four biophysical variables in the BPP score are fetal movement, fetal tone, fetal breathing movements (FBM) and AFV. The observations are made over a 30-minute period (although criteria are usually met in under 10 minutes) and a normal AFV is based on the largest vertical cord free pool being greater than 2 cm. In acute hypoxia FBM is one of the first variables to become abnormal, whereas AFV is a more chronic marker; of the various antenatal tests for fetal hypoxia, estimation of AFV probably has the lowest false-negative rate (i.e. least likely to miss fetal hypoxia).

79. A

In calculating the perinatal mortality rate (enumerator/denominator), the enumerator includes the number of stillborn babies (i.e. born with no signs of life at or after 24 completed weeks of gestation) and early perinatal deaths (babies dying during the first week of life), and the denominator is per 1000 total births. These babies are included in the calculation regardless of the cause of death. The neonatal period (first 4 weeks of life) is divided into early (first week) and late (subsequent 3 weeks). Perinatal mortality rates are the cornerstone for measuring obstetric care and are seen in the West as a measure of the quality of obstetric practice. Congenital malformations are one of the main causes of perinatal death, and sometimes what is called the 'corrected' perinatal mortality rate is calculated by excluding babies with fatal congenital anomalies.

80. ABCDE

The associations of perinatal mortality are many. The major ones are low birthweight, congenital abnormality and asphyxial events. In the first pregnancy there is a higher incidence of pre-eclampsia and of teenage pregnancy (many of which are concealed and unwanted). Increasing maternal age and parity result in the increase in maternal systemic disorders and obstetric illnesses. The most easily identifiable factor antenatally may be a previous pregnancy that ended in premature delivery, stillbirth or neonatal death.

81. BD

The fall in perinatal mortality rate seen in the 1970s is slowing and it is clear that the present rate is largely due to improved health of the population and neonatal services rather than to obstetric intervention. Marked regional variations seem to be explainable largely by the differences in low birthweight, although why the latter occurs is more difficult to discern. There is no evidence that routine ultrasonography has made any impact on perinatal mortality nationally, although the results from centres of excellence may suggest otherwise.

82. BD

In all animal species studied, birthweight is directly correlated with survival. Low birthweight alone is a better predictor of perinatal morbidity and mortality than gestational age alone, but for a given birthweight a greater gestational age is associated with decreased risk. Crude birthweight at term is a poor predictor of perinatal outcome as not all babies in the lower centile groups will be growth restricted. Similarly, not all babies over the traditional 2.5 kg at term have reached their full growth potential. The most important determinant of birthweight at term is gestational age.

83. BD

Rubella (or German measles, as it was recognized as a disease separate from measles by two German physicians) is usually a mild childhood illness. In pregnancy, however, rubella is very important as it can lead to congenital infection and abnormalities; up to 50% of fetuses are affected if the disease is contracted in the first trimester. The virus is carried in the nasopharynx and is spread by droplets. The diagnosis is usually made by serological tests, looking for either rubella-specific IgM (which does not persist for more than 1 month) or a rising titre of rubella antibodies.

84. AE

Parvovirus B19 is the cause of fifth disease, and, although usually asymptomatic, may present with the classical slapped cheek, fever, arthralgia and aplastic anaemia in those with an inherited haemolytic anaemia (e.g. sicklers). In the fetus, because of a predilection for the erythroid progenitor cells, it causes aplastic anaemia and fetal hydrops. Classically aplastic fetal crisis is antedated by a raised AFP level. Parvovirus does not cause any structural abnormality, nor is it a cause of IUGR.

85. BCD

In the general obstetric population the incidence of the lupus anticoagulant is about 1%, but in those with unexplained recurrent abortion it is probably about 20%. The risk to the fetus is clearly associated with antibody titres and women with systemic lupus erythematosus (SLE) who have very low levels of antibodies are probably at no excess risk. In the presence of significant antibody titres the fetal loss rate could be as high as 80%. Anti-Ro and anti-La antibodies are associated with congenital heart block. The lupus anticoagulant causes a prolongation of clotting time in vitro but paradoxically produces a thrombotic tendency in vivo.

86. AD

Probably the most important maternal risk factor in pre-eclampsia is primigravidity and, although secundiparae have a lower overall incidence, this is still at least ten times that of someone with a previously unaffected pregnancy. The risk of pre-eclampsia increases slightly with maternal age and the increase seen in the teenage years relates to parity rather than age. There is no association with social class or maternal weight. In fact, affected mothers tend to be lighter and shorter than average. Remember also that smokers tend to have a lower incidence of pre-eclampsia, but in smokers who do develop it, the outcome is worse than in non-smokers.

87. ACDE

ICD9 defines maternal death as: death of a woman while pregnant or within 42 days of pregnancy, irrespective of the duration and the site of the pregnancy, from any cause related to or aggravated by the pregnancy or its management but not from accidental or incidental causes (fortuitous).

Direct deaths are those resulting from obstetric complications of the pregnant state (pregnancy, labour and the puerperium), from interventions, omissions, incorrect treatment, or from a chain of events resulting from any of the above.

Indirect deaths are those resulting from previous existing disease or disease that developed during pregnancy and which was not due to direct causes, but which was aggravated by physiological effects of pregnancy.

There is underreporting. To improve coverage, ICD10 introduces a new category of 'pregnancy-related death' intended for use where the cause of death cannot be identified precisely.

From 1982 to 1990 in the UK, maternal death accounted for 0.7% of deaths in women aged 15–44 years.

88. DE

The responsibility for initiating enquiries rests with the Director of Public Health (DPH) of the district in which the woman was usually resident. Although the DPH receives death certificates for all residents, reference to pregnancy is not always included. Staff involved should notify the DPH, who arranges to collect all the information in a booklet and when completed by those who cared for the woman passes this to the Regional Obstetric Assessor. The Obstetric Assessor summarizes the case and gives an opinion in collaboration with the Regional Pathology Assessor and, where relevant, with the Regional Anaesthetic and Midwife (from 1994) Assessors. The completed booklet is forwarded to the Department of Health.

The Confidential Enquiries dealt with deaths in England and Wales from 1952. The first UK report covered the years 1985–1987. HM Coroner does not take part in the enquiries but many cases are reported to his/her office and autopsy may be carried out under his/her instruction.

No enquiry material or copies are kept by the DPH or Regional Assessors. At the Department of Health all identifying details are removed before assessment by the Central Assessors, and after preparation of the Report the enquiry forms are destroyed.

89. BE

Scottish death certificates contain a specific question on pregnancy but those used in England, Wales and Northern

Ireland do not. A recommendation in ICD10 is that death certificates should include such a question, otherwise there is a possibility of underreporting.

Since 1 January 1988, all deaths occurring within 6 months after pregnancy should be reported and those occurring between 6 and 12 months are included in the enquiries, if after discussion with the Regional Obstetric Assessor they are thought to be related to pregnancy. The Reports contain a separate chapter on Late Deaths, although these are not included in the mortality figures.

Substandard care is an opinion given by the authors of the Report and does not mean that death would have been avoided.

In the triennium 1985–1987 only one enquiry form from 265 known deaths was not completed, whereas from 1988 to 1990 14 of 339 were not available for analysis. There are various reasons for this shortfall. Late notification and initiation of the enquiries pose difficulties when staff involved have moved away, or case records and enquiry booklets are mislaid.

90. ABCD

The main direct cause of death was pulmonary embolism (30 cases). The second direct cause was hypertensive diseases of pregnancy (20 cases). Sadly, it was adjudged that care was substandard in 80% of these cases. Highlighted were delay in taking clinical decisions, poor control of blood pressure and a failure to recognize the seriousness of the case – often by staff at too junior a level. Ten of the 11 eclamptics had fits after admission to hospital. The setting up of regional teams of experts was advised on publication of the 1985–1987 report.

The estimated fatality rate per 1000 caesarean sections was 0.33 in the 1988–1990 report. An unplanned emergency caesarean operation is one in which clinical urgency overrides the standard full preoperative preparation. There was a marked reduction in deaths in these cases, probably because fewer rushed decisions were made.

No death associated with illegal abortion has been reported since 1981.

91. ACDE

Listeriosis occurs throughout pregnancy and should be considered when the mother has a pyrexial flu-like illness. Many cases, however, are asymptomatic. The fetus is usually affected, with intrauterine death occurring in up to 20% of cases.

92. AE

Twenty-four direct maternal deaths were due to pulmonary embolism: three occurred following operation for ectopic gestation, ten occurred antenatally, and 11 postnatally. Of these 11 postpartum deaths, eight were following caesarean section. The number of deaths from sepsis nearly doubled from the previous triennium and when deaths from postabortal sepsis are added to those from genital tract sepsis they amount to nearly 9% of direct maternal deaths.

Until the early 1980s anaesthesia was associated with more than one in ten direct maternal deaths. In this triennium (1988–1990) there were five deaths including one late death. Anaesthesia contributed to a further ten deaths. Substandard postoperative care was highlighted.

There were 19 deaths from ectopic pregnancy, with substandard care in seven cases. One death followed legal termination with no histological examination and in another case of uterine evacuation no action was taken following the report of scanty secretory endometrium and no evidence of pregnancy.

Although autopsy was carried out in 82% of all deaths known to the enquiry, 22% were considered to be inadequate and only 34% of high standard. It should be remembered that autopsy is unacceptable in some cultures.

93. AC

Glucose crosses the placenta by facilitated diffusion and stimulates fetal hyperinsulinaemia, which increases fetal oxygen demand. Lung maturation is delayed because hyperinsulinaemia hampers phospholipid synthesis. Hyperinsulinaemia also impedes the clearance of lung fluid immediately after delivery, resulting in transient tachypnoea. Caesarean delivery has this same ill effect.

The administration of β-mimetics has additional adverse effects in diabetics and may lead to hyperglycaemia, hyperinsulinaemia, hypocalcaemia, ketoacidosis and pulmonary oedema. Intensive monitoring is required when β-mimetics are used. Glucocorticoids have an additive effect. As for non-diabetics, folic acid should be given from 12 weeks before conception to 12 weeks' gestation.

Low-dose combined oral progestogens do not impair glucose tolerance. It is probably wiser to avoid monophasic ethinyloestradiol-norethisterone preparations because of reported changes in lipid-lipoprotein levels and to prescribe preparations containing levonorgestrel. Full investigation has not yet been carried out in the diabetic for preparations containing desogestrel, gestodene and norgestimate. Higher failure rates with copper IUCDs were reported in 1980s but since then no increased failure rate has been reported. The removal rate for infection is no different from that in non-diabetics.

94. BCD

The HbA_1C reflects diabetic control over the previous 4–8 weeks. The organs at risk of major malformation are formed by 9 weeks. The aim should be for tight control before conception and during the first 8 weeks (and, of course, during the rest of the pregnancy).

The incidence of cardiac malformations is increased fourfold compared with that in non-insulin-dependent diabetics. It is common practice for the mid-trimester anomaly scan to be repeated at 24 weeks if good views of the heart are not obtained. The incidence of anencephaly is increased fivefold.

More spontaneous abortions are associated with raised first trimester HbA_1C levels, probably as a result of poor glycaemic control around the time of conception rather than just before the abortion.

A study of hormonal dating of ovulation strongly suggested that the early growth delay demonstrated by ultrasonographic measurement in the late 1970s and 1980s was an artefact due to delayed ovulation.

95. ADE

About 25–30% require phototherapy. There is no increased incidence of anaemia. These infants are prone to polycythaemia – a response to increased erythropoietin resulting in an increased number of red blood cells that absorb glucose and may worsen hypoglycaemia.

There is no specific problem with potassium. Hypocalcaemia, which is related to the severity of the diabetes, occurs in 25–50% of these infants.

The temporary cardiomyopathy, an intraventricular septal hypertrophy, may lead to cardiac failure and is more common with hyperinsulinaemia, macrosomia and poor diabetic control.

Some 70% of infants with Erb's palsy recover completely and most of the remainder have some improvement.

96. CD

The 50th centile birthweight for boys is 4000 g at 42 weeks. A GTT performed for this weight indication is wasteful of resources for little pick-up. A more useful indication is for a previous birthweight greater than 4500 g at term or above the 97th centile for gestational age.

Almost half the cases of shoulder dystocia occur during the delivery of infants weighing less than 4000 g. Shoulder dystocia *per se* is not an indication for GTT; previous or current macrosomia is an indication.

Maternal weight greater than 100 kg and/or a body mass index above 30 are indications for a GTT. Excessive maternal weight gain during pregnancy increases the incidence of macrosomia and shoulder dystocia. Other indications include diabetes in a first-degree relative, previous unexplained stillbirth, previous glucose intolerance, glycosuria ++ on at least two occasions using BM urine strips.

97. ACD

Gestational diabetes includes diabetes unrecognized before pregnancy. The prevalence is increased 11-fold in women from the Indian subcontinent, eightfold in South-East Asian women, sixfold in Arab/Mediterranean women and threefold in black/Afro-Caribbean women compared with caucasians. Approximately 1 in 20 develop insulin-dependent diabetes within 5 years. Obesity is a risk factor. and weight loss should be actively encouraged after pregnancy as this lowers the incidence of diabetes developing. There is a need for follow-up. In these cases significant maternal hyperglycaemia does not occur until after organogenesis is complete.

98. ABDE

In a retrospective study the recurrence rate in the next pregnancy was 17 times the background rate amongst all deliveries. The incidence is increased when there is slow progress in late first stage, prolonged second stage and with mid-forceps deliveries.

Ultrasonography estimates give a value, but weight may vary by ±16–20%; thus a weight estimate of 4000 g means between

3200 and 4800 g. Realizing these limitations, it has recently been shown that formulae based on the abdominal circumference alone are almost as effective as more complicated ones.

Amongst other effects the McRoberts position with acutely flexed hips reduces the angle of inclination of the pelvic brim, straightens out the lumbar and lumbosacral lordosis, eliminates weight-bearing from the sacrum to allow the pelvis to achieve its maximum capacity as well as elevating the anterior shoulder. Suprapubic pressure is used almost universally but if inappropriately done in the midline, the anterior shoulder may become more jammed in the pelvic brim. Pressure should be applied in a more lateral direction, ideally to flex the shoulder girdle and decrease the bi-acromial diameter. Cephalic replacement with delivery by caesarean section is practised with success in some centres in the USA.

99. AE

The BPP score is similar to an intrauterine Apgar Score but maturation of fetal behavioural states is essential, so that interpretation is difficult before 26 weeks' gestation. Randomized trials have shown a reduction in perinatal mortality even when used on a selective basis. It is probably the optimal method of monitoring for fetal hypoxia in prolonged pregnancy with a false negative rate for mortality of 0.6 per 1000 within 1 week of a normal score. Because it depends on fetal behavioural state and biophysical variables, the BPP also assumes an intact CNS, and in the presence of an abnormal score the possibility of neurological dysfunction must be considered.

100. AB

Johann Christian Doppler (1805–1853) was born in Salzburg, the son of a master stonemason. As the Director of the Physical Institute and Professor of Experimental Physics at the Imperial Institute of Vienna, he submitted a paper in 1842 'On coloured light of double stars and some other heavenly bodies' to the Royal Bohemian Society of Learning. In 1845 the little known Dutch scientist D.H. Buys Ballot (1817–1890) challenged Doppler's theory and conducted the first Doppler sound experiment using three French horn players and the 1.30 pm train from Utrecht. He calculated the train's velocity to within 10%, based on the frequency shift perceived by his observers, but his findings were published in a journal for music lovers. Satomura (1959) used Doppler ultrasonography clinically to study peripheral vascular blood flow and in 1977 Fitzgerald and Drumm, two Dublin obstetricians, used the technique to study umbilical artery blood flow.

Continuous-wave devices are relatively inexpensive, blind using a pencil probe on the maternal abdomen and rely on a waveform pattern recognition to identify the vessel sampled. Pulsed-wave devices display a standard B-mode image on which a sample gate can be accurately placed. Because the angle of insonation is known in such devices, the true velocity can be calculated and, if the vessel diameter is measured, true volume flow measurements can be made. This is not possible with continuous-wave devices, although they provide flow velocity waveforms whose characteristics reflect the downstream vascular resistance. A high pass (i.e. one that blocks out information from low-frequency Doppler shifts filter (50 or 100 Hz) caused by vessel wall movement) is employed in some devices.

101. ABC

Umbilical artery waveform indices correlate well with tertiary stem villi count and with short-term morbidity in high-risk pregnancy but not with long-term outcome. There is conflicting published literature on whether or not the waveform indices in each twin's umbilical artery are discordant in twin–twin transfusion syndrome, and no consistent pattern has been observed.

102. ABD

During normal placental development 100–150 spiral arteries gradually become distended, tortuous, funnel-shaped vessels whose musculoelastic walls undergo two stages of 'trophoblast invasion'. The inner myometrial and decidual segments of the spiral arterioles lose their muscle coats during the first wave of trophoblast invasion at 10–12 weeks. During the second stage, at 12–16 weeks, the deeper myometrial segments are involved as far as the radial arteries. Abnormal uteroplacental waveforms thus reflect pathological spiral arteries that have retained their muscle coats, and they are classically described as having increased pulsatility and a notch in early diastole. The Pulsatility Index falls during normal pregnancy, although abnormal waveforms are predictors of pre-eclampsia and

IUGR. Because continuous-wave devices are blind, using a pencil probe on the maternal abdomen and relying on waveform pattern recognition to identify the vessel sampled, it has been suggested that accurate uteroplacental waveform analysis requires a pulsed Doppler device and ideally colour Doppler ultrasonography.

103. AC

Absent (AEDF) or Reversed End-Diastolic Flow (RDF) constitutes a significant fetal risk with a mortality rate of 40% and high perinatal morbidity. Progression from AEDF to reversed flow implies a higher risk of mortality. There is a significantly increased risk of major congenital structural abnormalities (21%) and abnormal karyotype (4%). When AEDF or RDF is suspected, the wall thump filter should be turned off; otherwise, low-frequency shifts will be removed by the filter (in this case those lower than 100 Hz).

104. BCD

The incidence of absent end-diastolic flow is low (0.03% at 28 weeks, 0.01% at 34 weeks in 2097 unselected pregnancies) and the outcome is varied. Whilst prompt intensive surveillance should be instituted, delivery should be for non-Doppler reasons after proper assessment of fetal health and normality. In such cases the RI = A-B/A, i.e. 1.0 (A will have a value for maximum systolic frequency shift and B is by definition zero).

105. CDE

In colour Doppler ultrasonography, a grey scale image is obtained on which Doppler information is displayed, using red to denote movement towards the transducer and blue movement away from it. Obviously such devices will display arterial and venous flow as either red or blue depending on the orientation of the transducer and the vessel. Colour intensity is related to the velocity of flow. The technique is of value in the diagnosis of congenital heart disease as flow dynamics may allude to structural defects (e.g. a small ventriculoseptal defect) not apparent on conventional B-mode imaging. In renal agenesis the lack of amniotic fluid reduces image quality severely and absence of renal artery blood flow is useful in confirming suspected renal agenesis.

106. AC

Power Doppler imaging produces a grey scale image on which Doppler information is superimposed. Unlike colour Doppler systems there is no directional information and colour intensity relates to the amplitude of the returning ultrasound beam, regardless of velocity (direction or speed). It is more sensitive than colour Doppler ultrasonography for identifying vessels with low-velocity blood flow. Aliasing is not reduced and, because there is no directional information, it cannot be used to study redistribution.

107. DE

Power output from colour Doppler devices is lower than that from pulsed-wave ones. High doses of ultrasound along the whole length of the pulsed-wave beam can cause significant heating at the bone-soft tissue interfaces. The area delineated by the sample gate is used to sample the returning waveform from that area, but has no effect on the transmitted beam. Cavitation and microbubble formation do not occur to any significant degree using obstetric pulsed-wave devices. A randomized trial of intensive versus minimal ultrasound imaging and Doppler studies was reported in 1995 and found a mean of 30 g reduction in the birthweight of the former group.

108. ACDE

Umbilical artery waveform indices are dimensionless and are independent of the angle of insonation. High pulsatility implies a high distal impedance in the placenta. The commonest indices are the Pulsatility Index (PI), Resistance or Pourcelot Index (RI) and the systole/diastole ratio (SD). The formula for each index is based on knowledge of the maximum frequency shift in systole (A), diastole (B) and the time-averaged mean (TAM) during the cardiac cycle, i.e.: PI = A-B/TAM, RI = A-B/A and SD = A/B. When there is zero diastolic flow or reversed flow, a value for PI can be calculated but SD is infinity and RI = 1.0.

109. BD

Whilst an AC measurement less than fifth centile is indicative of an SGA fetus, the term IUGR should be based on serial AC measurements showing a falling growth velocity or other features such as oligohydramnios or abnormal umbilical artery Doppler studies. The AC is related to fetal liver volume, which is reduced when stored glycogen is depleted as a response to gluconeogenesis in IUGR. Asymmetrical growth retardation (increased HC/AC) implies brain sparing or uteroplacental insufficiency-type growth retardation, whereas a symmetrical SGA fetus may be more likely to have an underlying chromosomal abnormality. Although weekly ultrasonographic surveillance may be appropriate in some high-risk pregnancies, serial biometry should be compared at 2-weekly intervals because of the errors in measurements such that true trend are not apparent if biometry is performed more frequently. HC and AC are the mainstay of serial growth assessment in the third trimester. BPD measurements are inaccurate and do not reflect fetal nutritional status as head sparing may occur even in severe IUGR.

110. ABCD

Classical type I or symmetrical IUGR may be due to chromosomal abnormality, fetal infection, ethnic and constitutional causes. Ideally correction should be made for maternal factors such as height, weight, parity and ethnic background, and this has been used to construct individual customized growth charts. The correct plane for the AC is a transverse section of the abdomen showing the spine and mid-region of the hepatic vein. In late pregnancy it is often difficult to obtain good HC measurements as the fetal head engages, and FL/AC ratios provide similar information to HC/AC ratios, with increased ratios suggestive of asymmetrical IUGR and uteroplacental insufficiency.

111. B

In twin–twin transfusion syndrome the discordancy is usually between the abdominal circumference measurements. A single late scan does have a high sensitivity for detection of small for dates fetuses. Linear measurements are accurate to about $\pm 10\%$ and measurements of circumference and area and estimated fetal weight are accurate to about $\pm 20\%$. Suspected fetal macrosomia may not always be confirmed on ultrasonography and estimates of fetal weight are most inaccurate at the extremes (i.e. in the small or large for gestational age fetus).

112. AC

Kick charts usually rely on the fact that most women will have felt ten separate episodes of movement within 12 hours of waking, and if not they are usually advised to contact their local maternity hospital to arrange for further fetal assessment. However, a randomized controlled trial involving over 68,000 pregnant women showed no effect on perinatal mortality when kick charts were employed on a routine, as opposed to a selective, basis. The false-positive rate was high, such that many low-risk fetuses (and their mothers) were referred for further assessment.

Placental site and breech position have not been shown to have a proven effect on the maternal perception of fetal movements. Furthermore, there is no evidence that fetal activity is reduced at term.

Maternal ingestion of glucose, and thus increased glucose supply to the fetus, may increase fetal activity; hence the common practice of giving the mother with reduced fetal movements a sugary drink.

113. BC

Antepartum classification by the International Federation of Obstetrics and Gynaecology (FIGO) is based on three categories as follows:

Normal: baseline 110–150 bpm, amplitude of baseline variability 5–25 bpm, absent decelerations except for mild decelerations of very short duration, presence of two or more accelerations during a 20-minute period.

Suspicious: Baseline of 150–170 bpm or 100–110 bpm, amplitude of baseline variability 5–10 bpm for more than 40 minutes, increased variability over 25 bpm (saltatory), absence of decelerations for more than 40 minutes, sporadic decelerations of any type unless severe.

Pathological: Baseline heart rate below 100 bpm or over 170 bpm, variability less than 5 bpm for more than 40 minutes, periodically recurring and repeated decelerations of any type, severe variable or late decelerations, or a sinusoidal pattern.

114. ABCDE

Late decelerations may be defined as a drop in the fetal heart rate with trough greater than 15 seconds after the peak of contraction. It is due to decreased uteroplacental blood flow, reduced oxygen transfer during a contraction, stimulation of the aortic arch chemoreceptors and increased parasympathetic activity with a consequent reduction in heart rate. The delay in fetal heart rate drop is due to time taken for blood to reach the aortic arch from the placenta.

Between contractions normal perfusion may result in normal baseline, variability, etc., suggesting adequate cerebral oxygenation but, if the fetus is already compromised, oxygen transfer during the contraction is not adequate for myocardial activity and direct myocardial depression occurs in addition to increased vagal activity. The rate of oxygen transfer between contractions may not be adequate to maintain oxygenation, resulting in reduced or absent variability, and eventually a baseline tachycardia occurs.

Causes of late deceleration are essentially anything that reduces uteroplacental blood flow, and include placental abruption, maternal hypotension, uterine hypertonia or hyperstimulation, maternal or pregnancy-related disease causing placental insufficiency (diabetes mellitus, pre-eclampsia, renal disease and the antiphospholipid antibody syndrome). Other conditions predisposing to or suggestive of existing fetal compromise include IUGR, prematurity, rhesus disease and twin–twin transfusion syndrome.

115. ABCE

Late decelerations are always associated with significant fetal hypoxia and management is directed towards increasing uteroplacental blood flow and oxygen delivery to fetus. These include changing maternal posture, stopping oxytocin infusion, assessment of maternal blood pressure and treatment of hypotension, and giving maternal oxygen by face mask. Fetal blood sampling should be performed unless variability is reduced or there is baseline tachycardia. In such cases delivery is more appropriate.

116. ABCDE

The contraction stress test (oxytocin challenge test) evaluates the fetal heart rate response to contractions induced by an intravenous bolus of Syntocinon. The procedure is dangerous to the fetus as severe fetal distress may be provoked. It is rarely indicated and should be performed only in the labour ward with full preparation for caesarean section. The false-negative rate is low (0.4 per 1000). All the comments about the non-stress test are correct. It is usually based on a 20-minute cardiotocogram, but may be extended to up to 40 minutes before failure to meet the criteria is defined as abnormal.

117. ABDE

Amniocentesis may be used to obtain amniotic fluid for karyotyping in women at increased risk of chromosomal abnormalities (i.e. those aged over 35 years, those who are screen positive on serum testing, those with a previously affected child). Women at high risk of having a child with spina bifida but in whom ultrasonographic imaging is limited by gross obesity may benefit from amniocentesis in which raised amniotic fluid α-fetoprotein and a double band for acetylcholinesterase may indicate an open neural tube defect. In rhesus disease, determination of bilirubin and lecithin/sphingomyelin ratios may be helpful in assessing the degree of haemolysis and lung maturity.

118. BCDE

Prenatal testing by amniocentesis and CVS are usually performed at 14–18 weeks and 10–12 weeks, with miscarriage risks of 0.5–1.0% and 1–2% respectively. There is also a small but recognized risk of limb reduction defects following CVS before 10 weeks and of postural limb defects following amniocentesis, especially if performed earlier than 14 weeks. There is also a suggestion that before 14 weeks (early) amniocentesis may result in a higher miscarriage risk than conventionally timed amniocentesis. Rhesus-negative mothers should receive 250 IU anti-D immunoglobulin after testing before 20 weeks and 500 IU after 20 weeks.

119. ABCE

Although fetal blood sampling had been described by Rodeck and Campbell using fetoscopy, Daffos first described in 1983 the technique of cordocentesis or PUBS (percutaneous umbilical blood sampling) in which a needle is inserted into the umbilical vein under ultrasonographic guidance. The sampling site is usually based on accessibility and sampling is usually performed after 18–20 weeks. The umbilical vein as it enters the placenta provides a useful target in that it is usually visible and is fixed. Other potential targets include the heart and the large hepatic vein that runs through the baby's liver. Most operators use a 20-gauge needle which has a polished echo-tip, allowing accurate visualization on ultrasonography. The procedure is carried out under direct ultrasonographic guidance but factors such as excessive fetal activity, failure to identify the cord insertion or a fetus overlying the cord insertion may prevent sampling altogether. Confirmation that the sample is fetal and pure is obtained by rapid analysis using a Coulter counter in the haematology laboratory to compare the sample blood with a previous sample taken from the mother (e.g. larger blood cells mean corpuscular volume (MCV) in the fetus, lower blood count (haemoglobin) than expected if sample diluted by amniotic fluid).

Patients do not require any analgesia for routine sampling but some centres advocate the use of antibiotics, local anaesthetic and sedation. Recent advances in DNA technology have actually reduced the indications for fetal blood sampling, with amniotic fluid and CVS samples being used where previously fetal blood was required, although the role in assessing fetal anaemia and haemolysis in rhesus disease remains unchallenged. Polymerase chain reaction for viral DNA in amniocentesis samples is the optimal method for assessing suspected intrauterine viral infection rather than fetal immunoglobulin levels in blood. In some IUGR pregnancies, fetal blood sampling is valuable for karyotyping, cord blood gas analysis and excluding viral infection. The main risks are similar to those of amniocentesis and CVS, and include infection, premature rupture of the membranes and fetal distress, although cord tamponade and exsanguination are specific risk factors. Obviously gestation at sampling, underlying fetal condition and operator skill are also important factors in determining outcome. Overall loss rates of about 2% are common in practice, but rates increase rapidly for sampling before 19 weeks when a loss rate of 5% and fetal distress (bradycardia) in 20% of cases may occur.

120. ABD

One of the most frequent causes of coccygodynia is damage to the sacrococcygeal ligament during vaginal delivery. Coccygectomy is used as a method of treatment, and is successful, but non-surgical measures are used as a first-line treatment. The pain of coccygodynia is often referred to the distribution of the pudendal nerve, which supplies the lower part of the vagina, the upper part being supplied by the autonomic nervous system via the uterovaginal plexus. Defaecation may be painful due to spasm of the posterior pelvic muscle, but normally micturition is not so affected.

121. CE

The most accurate time to determine amniocity and chorionicity is in the first trimester. Diamniotic dichorionic multiple pregnancies will show separate implantation sites and therefore for up to 10 weeks' gestation will show separate gestation sacs. After this gestation, separate placentas, female–male twin, thick separating membrane and peaking of the chorion at the edge of the abutting membranes indicate dichorionicity. The later in pregnancy twinning is diagnosed, the less accurate the ultrasonographic findings in determining chorionicity. Therefore early scanning is appropriate. Although scanning twins at 20 weeks' gestation is appropriate for screening for structural abnormalities, it is not performed at this gestation to determine the zygosity.

122. ACE

A raised maternal serum AFP level is found in many situations, the commonest cause being incorrect dating – the pregnancy being more advanced that determined by the last menstrual period – and multiple pregnancy. The level is increased with many 'open' abnormalities in which the integrity of the skin surface is broken. It is therefore not raised in many significant structural lesions. Abnormalities leading to impending or recent fetal demise will result in raised levels of AFP. Similarly recent placental bleeding causes the levels to increase.

123. BE

The maternal serum AFP will be normal in closed spina bifida, i.e. where the lesion is covered with skin. 95% of spina bifida cases show abnormalities in the head such as associated hydrocephalus, abnormal head shape (lemon-shape) and abnormal cerebellar shape (banana-shape), giving rise to the 'lemon and banana' sign. These findings form the Arnold-Chiari malformation. The cerebellum is abnormal in over 70% of cases. The only antenatal indicator of outcome is the level of the lesion. Prenatal movements in the lower limbs do not predict good limb function post delivery.

124. ABDE

Many structural abnormalities may form part of syndromes or be markers of a chromosomal abnormality. It is important to consider a karyotyping procedure when this information would alter the management of the pregnancy (e.g. a chromosomal abnormality previability which alters the prognosis of the structural lesion, or a lethal chromosomal abnormality viz. trisomy 18 when an operative delivery may not be appropriate).

125. C

In placenta praevia there are no published data to suggest that transvaginal ultrasonography is contraindicated. The improved definition, particularly in the posterior placenta, allows accurate identification of the leading placental edge in relation to the internal os. A fundal placenta may be associated with a succinturate lobe encroaching on the lower segment and causing bleeding. Placental abruption is a clinical diagnosis; ultrasonography does not have a role to play.

126. C

Movements of the fetal chest wall as observed by ultrasonography are termed 'fetal breathing movements'. They are primarily diaphragmatic and usually decrease in incidence within 72 hours of the spontaneous onset of labour, presumably due to increased fetal arterial prostaglandin E levels. They are one of the components of the biophysical profile score, and their presence is taken as an index of fetal health. They are periodic in nature and their absence, on the other hand, particularly over short observation intervals, does not necessarily imply fetal hypoxia.

127. ABDE

The most sensitive indicator of iron deficiency is the mean red cell volume (MCV), and it is the first red cell index to change in iron-deficiency anaemia of pregnancy. Total iron-binding capacity is raised in iron deficiency anaemia.

128. ABE

AFP is produced in the yolk sac, fetal liver and fetal gastrointestinal tract. Its concentration in fetal serum rises from the fourth week of gestation to peak at 12–14 weeks and then progressively falls towards term. Amniotic fluid AFP concentration runs parallel to fetal serum concentration but is approximately 150 times lower. Maternal serum AFP concentration is approximately 50,000 times lower and lags behind that in the fetus, rising from week 10 to week 32 and declining thereafter.

129. ACE

Because of mechanical elevation of the diaphragm in pregnancy there is change in the cardiac position and its electrical axis. There is usually a loud third heart sound in pregnancy, but this is an auscultatory finding and not detected on electrocardiography (ECG). The P-R interval is not changed.

130. BE

Male and female fetuses initially grow at the same rate until the 32nd week of gestation, when the male grows more rapidly. As early as 24–26 weeks the spaces between capillaries and airspaces in the fetal lungs are small enough to allow effective gas exchange in some babies. Also during this time the type II pneumocytes appear and have the ability to manufacture surfactants. Fetal blood glucose levels are about two-thirds of those of the mother, which facilitates glucose transfer. This is very important as over 90% of fetal energy requirements are obtained from glucose, hence it has been called a 'glucose-dependent parasite'.

131. BCE

From the beginning of pregnancy the production of luteinizing hormone is reduced as a result of negative feedback from the rising levels of oestrogen. Human chorionic gonadotrophin production peaks during the end of the first trimester and then drops to reach a plateau in the middle of the second trimester.

132. ACE

Oxytocin is synthesized in the nerve cells of the hypothalamic (supraoptic and paraventricular) nuclei and carried down the nerve axons in the pituitary stalk to the posterior lobe of the pituitary gland where it is secreted. Alcohol inhibits the secretion of oxytocin and, in the past, had been used as a tocolytic to reduce uterine contractions in preterm labour.

133. CE

During pregnancy oestrogen and prolactin synergize in producing breast growth, but oestrogen antagonizes the milk-producing effect of prolactin on the breast. After delivery of the placenta, there is an abrupt decline in the circulating levels of oestrogen, which leads to the initiation of lactation. In fact, oestrogen had been used in the past to suppress lactation (now obsolete because of the risk of thromboembolism). Normal breast growth and lactation can occur in dwarfs with congenital growth hormone deficiency. Progesterone does not inhibit lactation and is widely used for contraception in lactating women (e.g. progestogen-only oral pill and the long-acting injectable medroxyprogesterone).

134. AC

The following table and definitions illustrate the meaning of these commonly used terms.

	Women having the condition	Women not having the condition
screen-positive	true positive (a)	false positive (b)
screen-negative	false negative (c)	true negative (d)

Sensitivity (a/a+c) is the probability that the test will be positive if the condition is present. *Specificity* (d/b+d) is the probability that the test will be negative if the condition is absent. *Positive predictive value* (a/a+b) is the probability that the condition is present if the test is positive. *Negative predictive value* (d/c+d) is the probability that the condition is absent if the test is negative. The test will not have the same performance in the whole population because the incidence of condition (pre-eclampsia) is different between the study population (primigravid) and the whole population (primigravid and multigravid).

135. All answers are false

All these drugs may be prescribed safely during breastfeeding. It is also important to reassure the breastfeeding mother that the drugs will not adversely affect the baby as this may increase her compliance with the treatment.

136. BDE

Methyldopa is an α_2-agonist used widely in the treatment of hypertension during pregnancy. It acts, through its metabolite α-methylnoradrenaline, on the central α_2-receptors in the brain to reduce the sympathetic outflow. Methyldopa is slow acting and, therefore, not suitable for emergency treatment of hypertension when a more rapid hypotensive effect is required.

137. ACD

Oxytocin has about 5% of the antidiuretic effect of the hormone vasopressin and, in large doses, can lead to water intoxication and hyponatraemia. This is more likely if the drug is administered with large amounts of fluid.

138. DE

Although very large doses of metronidazole are teratogenic in rodents, there is no evidence that it is teratogenic in the human. Carbamazepine and all other commonly used anticonvulsant agents appear to be teratogenic, with a 5–10% incidence of fetal abnormality. In fact, epilepsy itself seems to be associated with a higher incidence of fetal abnormality, irrespective of drug treatment. Diethylstilboestrol (DES) leads to a wide spectrum of genital abnormalities in the fetus and is associated with vaginal adenosis and adenocarcinoma of the vagina in the female offspring.

139. BCD

Originally, ECV was almost always attempted before 36 weeks as it was thought to be rarely successful after that time. The effectiveness of this procedure remained controversial and randomized controlled trials had failed to demonstrate any effect on the breech birth, caesarean section rates or perinatal outcome. However, more recent randomized controlled trials of ECV *at term* show reduction of breech presentation at birth and almost halving of the caesarean section rate. The risk of ECV to the mother is small and is mainly due to the drugs used to facilitate the procedure and to the rare risk of placental abruption. However, the risk to the fetus is greater, especially if general anaesthesia is used.

140. ABE

Throughout the world the incidence of twin birth varies considerably. Most of the geographical variation in twinning rates is considered to be due to variation in the dizygotic twinning rate, with the monozygotic twinning rate being constant at around 3.5 per 1000 maternities. The prevalence of conjoint twins resulting from very late and imperfect division of the embryo has been quoted at one in 200 monozygotic twins, with increased risk in triplet pregnancy.

141. ABDE

Because of the extensive blood supply to the pelvic organs and the vascular pedicles created in routine operations, the risk of postoperative bleeding is always present. The majority of cases occur within the first 48 hours and are caused usually by a pedicle becoming freed from its ligature. The bleeding may be clinically obvious as vaginal bleeding. However, in most cases it is intraperitoneal. Tachycardia, hypotension, diminished urine output and increased urine specific gravity are all signs suggestive of the possibility of intra-abdominal haemorrhage. Patients who have had significant intraoperative haemorrhage and a large volume of blood replacement may have depleted coagulation factors and may be bleeding from an unrecognized coagulopathy.

142. ABE

The duration of labour before caesarean section is probably the most significant risk factor. The longer the duration of labour, the higher the risk regardless of the condition of the membranes. Rupture of membranes is a very significant factor and the risk is directly proportional to the duration of membrane rupture before the operation. Women having general anaesthesia have been shown to be at higher risk of postoperative infection than those receiving regional analgesia. However, this appears to be due mainly to the characteristics of the women having general anaesthesia, the majority of whom are urgent cases, often delivered after prolonged duration of labour and after several vaginal examinations. The number of vaginal examinations following rupture of membranes correlates closely with the risk of endometritis and wound infection. The majority of studies addressing the risk of maternal infection as a result of using internal fetal monitoring have concluded that no greater risk is incurred by this method.

143. ABD

Erb's palsy, presenting with limited abduction, pronation and internal rotation of the arm, is the largely self-limiting result of traction on the upper roots (C4, C5, C6) of the brachial plexus during delivery. No specific therapy is needed unless there is lack of spontaneous recovery over several weeks. Shoulder dystocia and rotation forceps deliveries are regularly associated with this complication. The diaphragm is supplied by the same nerve roots and ipsilateral diaphragmatic paralysis can occur.

144. BCE

Physiological jaundice in the newborn arises after 48 hours, has resolved after about 10 days, and results from an increased level of unconjugated (lipophilic) bilirubin in blood and tissues. It is exaggerated by bruising or excessive red cell breakdown. Levels of conjugated bilirubin (bilirubin mono- or di-glucuronide) are very low or absent as these chemicals are excreted by the healthy liver through the biliary tract to the gut.

Conjugated hyperbilirubinaemia is an association of liver disorder or disease including metabolic problems such as galactosaemia or structural abnormalities such as biliary atresia. Urine will be dark because of the presence of bilirubin, whereas stools may be pale because of its absence.

145. CDE

Establishment of airway and circulation are the prime aims of neonatal resuscitation, required when spontaneous effective ventilation is not established. This may be because of hypoxia-ischaemia, drug-induced depression, trauma or congenital anomaly. The Apgar score at 10 minutes and beyond provides one index of long-term outcome if measured in a baby having effective resuscitation; a low 1-minute Apgar score provides a description of the baby at that stage.

Resuscitation equipment has a manometric blow-off valve, usually set at a pressure of 20–30 cmH_2O to reduce lung damage from positive-pressure lung inflation. If there is suspicion of meconium in major airways, an attempt should be made to aspirate this before positive pressures are applied.

146. ABCD

These form part of the UNICEF/WHO statement recommended to maternity services as 'ten steps to successful breastfeeding', and are of proven benefit. Other important areas for maternity facilities include having a written and well-circulated policy on breastfeeding; training staff to implement this; educating all pregnant women on the benefits of breastfeeding; showing mothers how to lactate, even if they are separated from their infants; giving newborns no food or drink other than breast milk unless medically indicated; and fostering community support groups.

147. ABCD

Babies whose stores of glycogen have been exhausted during labour, by the stresses of maintaining core temperature or by infection are at risk of hypoglycaemia. Growth-restricted babies, preterm babies and babies who cannot be fed (for instance because of tachypnoea) are also at risk. Infants of diabetic mothers, including gestational diabetics, have a different problem, that of temporary excessive insulin secretion secondary to prenatal hyperstimulation. At-risk infants are usually screened by regular whole blood glucose testing, and fed early and regularly on milk.

148. BCE

Respiratory distress syndrome (RDS) occurs because of a relative deficiency of surfactants in the lung. The development of mature lung function is promoted by antenatal administration of steroids to mothers between 1 and 7 days before delivery. Affected babies can be helped by early instillation of surfactant intratracheally. RDS is not directly affected by delivery route, although asphyxia or hypothermia will inhibit natural surfactant production. RDS (which presents clinically within 4 hours of birth) remains an important association of morbidity and mortality in neonates both directly and through its association with intracranial disorders, patent ductus arteriosus, infection and chronic lung disease.

149. CD

Congenital diaphragmatic hernia is often one component of a multisystem disorder leading to an overall survival rate of less than 20% in obstetric-based series. The main predictor of outcome is lung function, the degree of pulmonary hypoplasia correlating poorly with the presence of particular organs or overall size of the defect. Although predominantly left sided, leading to herniation of stomach and intestines and apparent dextrocardia, small right-sided defects can occur which are blocked by the liver and may be found coincidentally on chest radiography. At birth, cardinal clinical signs would be a scaphoid abdomen, apparent dextrocardia, absence of breath sounds on the left and respiratory distress with cyanosis.

150. BCDE

Although in vitro studies have shown that many drugs (including ampicillin) interfere with bilirubin-albumin binding, this effect has been shown to be important in vivo only in the case of sulphonamides.

151. ABD

The term neonate has reduced levels of proteins S and C; clotting factors II, VII, IX and X; and antithrombin III. It has relatively high haematocrit, blood viscosity and levels of clotting factors V and VIII.

152. C

'A' is a sex-linked condition which usually presents in the first decade of life. 'B' and 'D' are autosomal dominant conditions, whereas 'C' is autosomal recessive and usually presents in utero. 'E' has a multifactorial background and may have a recurrence rate of 2–3%.

153. BCE

Haemophilia is carried through the female so an affected father will not pass the condition to his son but any daughters will be at risk of being carriers. An affected cousin on the mother's side indicates that all women (i.e. aunts) are at risk of being carriers so their male offspring will be at risk. A girl in an affected family who has Turner's syndrome will be at risk because she has a single X chromosome. Down's syndrome does not carry any added risk of haemophilia. If the mother is a carrier and the father is affected then the offspring will have the probability of being one carrier female, one normal and one affected male, and one affected female.

154. BCE

Huntington's disease presents in the fourth decade of life and is autosomal dominant. Meckel-Gruber syndrome comprises polydactyly, encephalocele and infantile polycystic renal disease. Joubert's syndrome comprises aplasia or hypoplasia of the cerebellar vermis. Achondroplasia is autosomal dominant.

155. CDE

Triploid cells contain three sets of the haploid number of chromosomes, (i.e. 69). Triploidy is a common finding in spontaneously aborted products of conception but rare in live-born children. Survival beyond the early neonatal period occurs only in children who are mosaics – with diploid and triploid cells. Most cases are due to dispermy or to fertilization by diploid sperm – such a double paternal contribution can lead to partial hydatidiform changes in the placenta. When triploidy results from an additional set of maternal chromosomes, the placenta is usually small. Complete triploidy is associated with severe IUGR, with relative preservation of head growth at the expense of a small trunk.

156. AE

'Gene tracking' (i.e. following the inheritance of a disease gene through a family) has to be used when the mutation causing the disease in a particular family is unknown, or when the chromosomal location of a disease is known but the gene responsible has not yet been isolated. Different types of DNA sequence variants can be used to demonstrate 'linkage' of a DNA marker with the disease locus – this allows diagnosis without knowledge of the biochemical defect, and in tissues where the gene is not usually expressed. The error rate is related to the risk of recombination between the DNA marker and the disease locus, and is lowest when two markers (one on each side of the gene, 'flanking markers') or a marker within the gene itself are used. To use gene tracking for prenatal diagnosis in a recessive disorder, the marker associated with the recessive gene in each of the parents must be identified by determining the DNA marker pattern of an affected child. A child with a recessive disorder must have inherited two copies of the disease gene, one from each parent The DNA marker pattern of the child will therefore determine which of the marker alleles in each parent is being inherited with the recessive disease. A fetus inheriting the same marker pattern as the affected child will be predicted to be affected, assuming absence of recombination and no genetic heterogeneity. Therefore, DNA samples from at least the parents and an affected child are needed. Gene tracking can be used only when DNA markers closely linked to the gene have already been identified.

157. ABCDE

A dominant condition is one that is expressed in the heterozygote; only one copy of the abnormal gene is required for expression. Therefore, if the mutation causing the disease in a particular family had been identified, accurate diagnosis would be possible for any family members who wished it (after suitable counselling) by testing directly for the presence of the mutation. In those families where gene tracking has to be used (i.e. a pathological mutation has not been identified) or where markers are identified but the gene has not yet been isolated, DNA will be required from several members to establish the DNA marker variant that is being inherited with the disease gene in that family. In some families it is not possible to track the gene because the DNA markers being inherited with the disease and normal genes give the same DNA marker pattern – they are 'uninformative'. If genes at different chromosomal locations can cause the disease (genetic heterogeneity), gene tracking using the DNA marker associated with only one locus will obviously give inaccurate results in some families.

158. BD

A small additional chromosome (known as a marker chromosome) presents a very difficult counselling problem. If the marker chromosome is present in one of the parents, it is unlikely that it will be of significance to the fetus. If it is a *de novo* finding, however, some studies give a risk of up to 15% that the fetus will be phenotypically abnormal. The size of the marker does not necessarily correlate with its clinical significance: the chromosomal region (and hence the genes) from which the marker is derived is most important. Some markers contain only heterochromatin (which is considered inactive). A small marker chromosome comprised entirely of euchromatin would give cause for concern. Although chromosome anomalies are often associated with congenital malformations, a normal ultrasonographic scan cannot completely eliminate the risk of mental retardation; prospective studies are underway to try to determine this risk.

159. ABCE

Apparent chromosomal mosaicism is found in about 1% of chorionic villus samples. Maternal cell contamination is more likely with cultured cells than with direct preparations. If the mosaicism is limited to a portion of the placenta (confined placental mosaicism), this is caused by an error in mitosis in the trophoblast, the fetus having normal chromosomes. It may be necessary to repeat fetal karyotyping on additional tissues (amniotic fluid cells or fetal blood, for instance) to resolve the uncertainty. It can be impossible to predict the phenotypic outcome when mosaicism is found; the effect of the abnormal karyotype depends on the number of cells with this karyotype and on their tissue and organ distributions. Usually several cell cultures are established to reduce the chance of cultural artefacts; if mosaicism is found in only one culture it is usually considered not to be a true reflection of the fetal karyotype. Counselling can be difficult but it is important that karyotyping is performed on the placenta or blood after delivery for confirmation of the findings.

160. BD

Fertility is normal in the XYY syndrome which is found in 1 in 1000 males in newborn surveys. Physical appearance is normal and stature usually above average. Intelligence may be mildly impaired compared with normal. The additional Y chromosome must arise as a result of non-disjunction in paternal meiosis II or as a postzygotic event. Gynaecomastia occurs in Klinefelter's syndrome (47,XXY), not 47,XYY.

161. ABCD

Indications for chromosome analysis include multiple congenital abnormalities, unexplained learning difficulties, sexual ambiguity or abnormality in sexual development, recurrent miscarriage, unexplained stillbirth, and malignancy and chromosome breakage syndromes. Chromosome abnormalities account for 50% of all spontaneous miscarriages and are present in 0.5–1% of newborn. Chromosome anomalies disrupting the retinoblastoma gene at 13q can provide the 'first hit' in the two-step pathogenesis of retinoblastoma. In 3–6% of couples with three or more pregnancy losses, one partner is found to carry a balanced translocation. Chromosome analysis should be amongst the first investigations undertaken in a newborn with ambiguous genitalia to aid assignment of the sex of rearing, and to warn of the potentially life-threatening diagnosis of salt-losing congenital adrenal hypoplasia.

162. All are false

Although he is the only affected person in his family, one cannot assume that his children have a low risk of inheriting any of the conditions because all can be inherited as autosomal dominant traits. Other members of the family may have the conditions but the diagnosis not yet made because of variation in expression (e.g. dominant retinitis pigmentosa). It is possible that his disease could be the result of a new mutation. Further family studies and investigations are required before accurate genetic information can be given. 'A', 'D' and 'E' can also be inherited as autosomal recessive and X-linked recessive conditions.

163. ABD

Genetic counselling is the process by which patients or relatives at risk of a disorder that may be hereditary are given information about the consequences of the disorder, the probability of developing and transmitting it, and the ways in which it may be prevented or ameliorated. Steps in genetic counselling include diagnosis (through history, examination, investigations), risk assessment, explanation and discussion of options, and long-term contact and support. The purpose is to give the family the information necessary to arrive at their own informed decision having considered all the choices open to them. Whatever the personal views of the counsellor, families are entitled to receive information about all options.

164. ACE

A detailed family tree enables a pattern of inheritance to be inferred where several affected members are present. The family history may help confirm a diagnosis or show whether the family structure would be suitable for gene tracking. Some autosomal conditions are more common in certain ethnic groups, so information about the family background may be important for screening for carrier status. A 'negative' family history would be expected in most couples who have babies with multiple congenital anomalies and so will not necessarily give warning of an increased risk. A negative family history in the families of cousins marrying does not rule out the possibility of their being at increased risk of being carriers for the same autosomal recessive condition.

165. CDE

A balanced reciprocal translocation originates from breaks having occurred in each of two chromosomes (during meiosis) and exchange of segments between them. Each of the derivative chromosomes contains material from both of the original chromosomes. The translocation is said to be 'balanced' when there is no loss or gain of genetic material and consequently there are no phenotypic effects in a carrier (with the exception of extremely rare cases in which a breakpoint damages an important functional gene). The incidence is approximately 1 in 500; the majority of translocation carriers have inherited the translocation from a parent. Usually the chromosome number remains at 46 and the breakpoints are unique to an individual family. If a child inherits the unbalanced form of the translocation, this can cause multiple abnormalities and learning disabilities, and so carriers of translocations should be offered prenatal diagnosis. An offer to test other family members for carrier status should be made: the regional clinical genetics service would usually organize this.

166. B

Chromosomal mosaicism for 45,X/46,XY results in a normal male phenotype in the majority of cases, only a small proportion having ambiguous or female external genitalia. This is not a likely explanation for the finding in this question. Androgen insensitivity (testicular feminization syndrome) coded by a gene on the X chromosome has a normal male karyotype with an essentially normal female phenotype. The vagina ends blindly and the uterus and fallopian tubes are absent. Testes are located in the abdomen or in the inguinal canal. In true hermaphroditism (which is extremely rare) an individual has both testicular and ovarian tissue, often in association with ambiguous genitalia. Most patients with true hermaphroditism have 46,XX karyotype with the paternally derived X chromosome carrying Y chromosome-specific DNA sequences. The most likely explanations also include the possibility of a mix-up of samples.

167. BDE

Although there is only one boy affected with Duchenne muscular dystrophy in this family, his female relatives could still be at high risk of being carriers of this X-linked condition. There is a 1 in 3 chance that his condition is due to a new mutation (his female relatives, including his mother would then not be at risk of being carriers). However, there is a risk of 2 in 3 that the mother of an isolated case is a carrier; therefore his sister who is pregnant has a 1 in 3 chance of being a carrier. Although creatine kinase estimation can be helpful in carrier detection, it is unreliable in pregnancy. This woman requires an urgent genetic opinion to assess her risk on the basis of the pedigree structure, and also to determine whether her brother has had DNA studies of the dystrophic gene. If he has a deletion of the dystrophic gene, for instance, his sister could be offered fetal sexing and testing for this deletion without having to determine her carrier status until after the pregnancy. Where there are several affected boys in a family, it may be possible to say with certainty from the pedigree which women must be carriers.

168. ABCDE

Cystic fibrosis (CF) is an autosomal recessive condition (the gene is located on chromosome 7). At conception, a child of two carriers of CF has a 1 in 4 chance of being affected, a 1 in 2 chance of being a carrier and a 1 in 4 chance of not having inherited a CF gene. In this case, the patient's partner is not affected: therefore he has a 2 in 3 chance of being a carrier. She has the population carrier risk of 1 in 20 as she has no family history of CF. It is possible to offer DNA testing for the common mutations (including delta F508). If none of these common mutations is found in the patient or her partner, their carrier risks will fall substantially. However, there would remain a small probability that both could be carriers of one of the rare mutations so that their having an affected child cannot be completely excluded, although this is unlikely. Prenatal diagnosis and carrier testing is extremely accurate when the precise mutations in a family have been identified.

169. ABCDE

Some dominant disorders (e.g. neurofibromatosis, tuberous sclerosis) can affect family members who have inherited the gene in widely different ways: some may have severe manifestations whereas others may have such minor manifestations that the diagnosis is not made until they are examined carefully. This is 'variation in expression' and is common in autosomal dominant disorders. 'Lack of penetrance' of a gene occurs when a family member shows no signs whatsoever of a dominant disorder but must have the gene, as he or she has an affected parent and child. This is relatively rare, but is recognized in retinoblastoma. New mutations for some dominant disorders increase with increasing paternal age. Sometimes environmental factors can cause a malformation that can also be caused by a genetic defect – a 'phenocopy'. Mistaken paternity could also be the explanation for the child's anomaly. The risks to future children vary widely depending on the cause: in this family, variation in expression was the reason as minor signs were found on radiography of the man's hands.

170. BDE

Galactosaemia is autosomal recessive and haemophilia is X-linked recessive.

171. ACE

Nuclear chromatin (Barr body) represents an inactivated X chromosome, which may be maternal or paternal in origin. It appears early, probably around the time of implantation. During interphase the number of Barr bodies present in a nucleus is one less than the number of X chromosomes present. In androgen insensitivity syndrome (46,XY) there are no Barr bodies, and in a female with Down's syndrome (47,XX,+21) there is one.

172. BE

As the number of Barr bodies present in a nucleus is one less than the number of X chromosomes present, there are no Barr bodies in Turner's syndrome. During early intrauterine development there is a normal number of germ cells. These germ cells, however, fail to surround themselves with granulosa cells during development, do not form follicles and are destroyed before term.

173. ABE

There is an internationally agreed chromosomal nomenclature. The chromosomal complement is designated by: (1) the total number of chromosomes, (2) the sex chromosome complement, and (3) any specific abnormality. 't' refers to translocation, 'del' to deletion, 'i' to isochromosome, and 'r' to ring chromosome. A karyotype containing additional or missing autosomes is signified by '+' and '−' respectively, followed by the number of the chromosome affected (e.g. female trisomy 21: 47,XX,+21). The chromosome with the lower number is recorded first, but if a sex chromosome is involved this comes first. 'p' refers to the short arm and 'q' refers to the long arm. Numbers following 'p' or 'q' refer to the band affected. In the example given in the question, the total number is 46 (normal) and the sex chromosomes are XX (female phenotype). There is translocation between band 21 on the short arm of chromosome X and band 23 on the long arm of chromosome 7.

174. ABCD

Down's syndrome is the commonest inherited cause of learning disability, with an incidence of about 1 in 700 live births, the second commonest cause being fragile X syndrome (1 in 1000). In about 5% of cases, Down's syndrome results from chromosomal translocation, but the question specified trisomy 21 (95% of cases), which results from non-disjunction.

175. ABDE

In translocation the chromosomes become broken (during meiosis or mitosis) and the resulting fragments become joined to other chromosomes. Reciprocal translocation involves an exchange of material between two non-homologous chromosomes. In balanced translocation there is normal number of chromosomes and amount of genetic material but this material is rearranged. These individuals are phenotypically normal, but have an increased risk of producing offspring with an abnormal amount of genetic material (unbalanced translocation).

176. ABCE

Between 30 and 40% of singletons present by the breech at 20–25 weeks and 15% at 32 weeks; premature babies comprise about 25% of babies born breech. By 34 weeks most would have undergone spontaneous version to cephalic presentation. Factors that may prevent spontaneous version include multiple pregnancy, oligohydramnios, polyhydramnios, hydrocephaly, intrauterine death, placenta praevia, cornual placenta (present in about 70% of term breech cases compared with 5% of controls) and congenital uterine abnormalities, when there is usually recurrence of breech presentation in subsequent pregnancies. In a multipara with a breech presentation, there is a 14% incidence of previous breech delivery.

177. BDE

Prematurity (and not post-term pregnancy) is present in 25% of cases of face presentation. Other associated factors are multiparity, multiple pregnancy, the presence of several loops of cord around the fetal neck, fetal goitre, polyhydramnios, pelvic tumour, bicornuate uterus and placenta praevia. Anencephaly is present in about 10% of cases, but this proportion would be higher if it was not for the fact that most anencephalic fetuses are now detected and terminated antenatally. Dolichocephaly (narrow elongated head) is usually a result of face delivery and not its cause.

178. ACD

Transverse or oblique lie occurs in about 1 in 300 cases. Predisposing factors include multiparity, pendulous abdomen, pelvic tumours, contracted pelvis, intrauterine death, prematurity, multiple pregnancy, placenta praevia, polyhydramnios and congenital uterine abnormalities. There is associated cord prolapse in about 15% of cases. Transverse lie of the second twin should be dealt with by internal podalic version and breech extraction performed by an experienced operator.

179. CE

Maternal rubella infection in the first trimester is associated with an affected fetus in 10–50% of cases, with the higher figures found in the earliest gestations. Each year in the UK there are about 20 reported cases of newborn babies with congenital rubella syndrome and between 100 and 200 cases of legal abortion for rubella infection during pregnancy. About 2–3% of pregnant women in the UK are susceptible (non-immune) to rubella. The RCOG recommends that women should be screened for rubella antibody in every pregnancy, irrespective of an earlier positive result or history of immunization. This is because the earlier test could have been with the older haemagglutination inhibition method that, unlike the newer radial haemolysis method, can give rise to so-called 'false positives'. Also the possibilities of vaccine failure (2–5% of cases), or a clerical or technical error with the original test warrant retesting.

A person infected with rubella is infectious from 7 days before to 7 days after the appearance of the rash, and IgM (the marker of current or recent infection) takes up to 21 days to appear in the blood of a new case.

The risk of fetal infection in case of inadvertent rubella immunization during pregnancy is thought to be very small. However, there are reported cases of women having an abortion following such an incident where the rubella virus has been isolated from fetal tissue.

180. BD

Secondary postpartum haemorrhage, by definition, may occur at any time between the first postnatal day and the sixth week of the puerperium. However, the commonest time for this presentation is the second week. Most cases are mild and settle down on conservative management, which should include antibiotics if there is any suspicion of infection as endometritis might be contributory. Ultrasonography will usually show echogenic uterine contents suggestive of retained products. However, this is more likely to indicate intrauterine blood, which is manifesting externally as bleeding. In the absence of heavy bleeding or an open cervical os on digital examination, surgical evacuation should not be the first line of management.

181. ABE

There are wide geographical variations in the incidence of intrahepatic cholestasis of pregnancy (IHCP). In Scandinavian countries, Canada, Chile, Poland, Australia and China, an incidence of up to 2% has been reported. The exact incidence in the UK is unknown, but seems to be less than 2%. IHCP usually presents in the third trimester with generalized pruritus, which may become progressively severe and is typically relieved within 48 hours of delivery. In some instances no further symptoms will develop; the so-called 'pruritus gravidarum'. More typically, jaundice develops 2–4 weeks after the onset of pruritus and also disappears rapidly postpartum. Serum levels of bile acids are often raised (from 10- to 100-fold), with a mild increase in the level of liver enzymes. Several studies have shown that serum levels of bile acids correlate with the severity of pruritus and the increased risk of fetal problems. These problems include preterm labour, fetal distress, meconium staining and intrauterine death.

182. ABCDE

The incidence of pre-eclampsia is about 6% in a first pregnancy. It affects about 2% of all second pregnancies, rising to 12% if the first pregnancy was affected and falling to 0.7% if the first pregnancy was a singleton normotensive pregnancy. Recurrent pre-eclampsia should heighten the index of suspicion for an underlying cause such as a renal or autoimmune disorder. Cholestasis of pregnancy is reported to recur in up to 45% of subsequent pregnancies, and may also recur if the woman takes the combined oral contraceptive pill. Preterm labour has a recurrence rate of 20–25%, compared with a background incidence of about 6%. Placenta praevia affects 0.5% of pregnancies, with a recurrence rate of up to 4–8% in subsequent pregnancies. Placental abruption affects 0.5–3% of pregnancies, with a recurrence rate of up to 6%; and in more than half of these cases the recurrence is more severe than the original episode.

183. B

Doppler scanning is accurate in detecting thrombosis in the leg veins (femoral and below), but not in pelvic veins. The fetal radiation doses of different imaging investigations are as follows: V/Q scan, 0.05 rad; CT pelvimetry, 0.08 rad; radiographic contrast venography, 0.5 rad; and radiographic pelvimetry, 0.5–1.1 rad, depending on how many views are taken. It is estimated that in utero exposure in excess of 5 rad will predispose to some types of childhood malignancy, but no dose – however small – should be considered totally safe, and the benefits should be balanced against the potential risks.

3

Gynaecological Oncology

Questions

184. Carcinoma of the vulva:

A. is increasing in incidence in the Western world.
B. is a common sequelae of vulval intraepithelial neoplasia.
C. is rarely found in association with maturation disorders.
D. is associated with other lower genital tract squamous cancers.
E. can develop from condyloma accuminatum.

185. In the treatment of squamous cell carcinoma of the vulva:

A. stage I lateralized lesions should be treated by radical vulvectomy and bilateral inguinal lymphadenectomy.
B. a 2-cm clitoral lesion is appropriately managed by wide local excision and bilateral groin node dissection through separate groin incisions.
C. the groin nodes need not be removed in superficially invasive localized lesions.
D. if, on frozen section, the deep femoral node is found to be involved, the iliac nodes should be resected.
E. simple vulvectomy is the most appropriate treatment in elderly patients.

186. In vulval intraepithelial neoplasia (VIN):

A. bowenoid dysplasia is more likely to progress to carcinoma than basaloid dysplasia.
B. if there is dysplasia elsewhere in the lower genital tract (multicentric disease), the risk of progression to invasion is higher.
C. the posterior fourchette is the most common site.
D. laser treatment should be performed to a depth of at least 5 mm.
E. topical 5-fluorouracil (5-FU) has been shown to be the most effective treatment.

187. Cervical cancer:

A. is the second most common cancer in the world.
B. in the UK, is increasing in women aged less than 40 years.
C. requires pelvic lymphadenectomy to assess the FIGO stage.
D. is not amenable to surgical treatment if the stage is IVa.
E. is not sensitive to radiotherapy if it is an adenocarcinoma.

188. In the treatment of cervical cancer, radiotherapy:

A. is usually curative in doses of 30 Gy.
B. improves survival if patients are pretreated with chemotherapy.
C. it is important to extend the treatment field to include the para-aortic lymph nodes.
D. can cause diarrhoea during treatment.
E. may result in second pelvic primaries up to 20 years after treatment.

189. Serum α-fetoprotein (AFP) concentration is a clinically useful tumour marker for:

A. Brenner tumours of the ovary.
B. mucinous cystadenocarcinoma of the ovary.
C. endodermal sinus tumours of the ovary.
D. granulosa cell tumours.
E. arrhenoblastoma.

190. In patients treated with cisplatin:
A. alopecia almost always occurs.
B. the usual dose is 250 mg per m^2 body surface area.
C. antiemetics are required.
D. intravenous hydration during treatment is required.
E. peripheral neuropathy is a late side-effect.

191. Groin lymph node dissection is not required in the following vulval cancers:
A. melanoma penetrating to a depth of 10 mm.
B. squamous cancer invading to a depth of 6 mm.
C. basal cell carcinoma.
D. verrucous carcinoma.
E. superficially invasive (up to 1 mm) squamous cancer.

192. With regard to endometrial carcinoma:
A. the incidence is increasing.
B. up to 25% of cases occur in premenopausal women.
C. there is a worse prognosis if histological examination shows squamous metaplasia.
D. adenomatous hyperplasia has a greater malignant potential than atypical hyperplasia.
E. stage Ic disease implies myometrial involvement to beyond the inner third of the myometrium.

193. Stage Ia1 cervical cancer:
A. is defined as stromal invasion of no more than 3 mm and a maximum width of 7 mm.
B. applies to both squamous and glandular lesions.
C. usually presents as a result of postcoital or postmenopausal bleeding.
D. is associated with pelvic lymph node metastasis in less than 2% of cases.
E. with stage Ia2 accounts for approximately 20% of all invasive cervical cancer.

194. Granulosa cell tumours of the ovary:
- **A.** account for about 70% of all stromal ovarian tumours.
- **B.** can be benign.
- **C.** secrete oestrogen in about one-quarter of cases.
- **D.** are associated with endometrial carcinoma in 10% of cases.
- **E.** usually present in an advanced stage.

195. The prognosis of patients with endometrial carcinoma is worse:
- **A.** in the elderly.
- **B.** when there is cervical involvement.
- **C.** when the tumour is poorly differentiated
- **D.** in diabetics.
- **E.** in women with hypertension.

196. The following are colposcopic features suggestive of early invasion:
- **A.** acetowhite epithelium.
- **B.** surface contour changes.
- **C.** mosaicism.
- **D.** atypical vessels.
- **E.** leucoplakia.

197. With regard to lymph node metastases in cervical cancer:
- **A.** 20% of patients with clinical stage Ib (Ib1 and Ib2) will have positive pelvic lymph nodes.
- **B.** 80% of patients with stage IVa disease will have involved pelvic lymph nodes.
- **C.** 20% of patients with stage IIb will have positive para-aortic lymph nodes.
- **D.** computed tomography has an accuracy in excess of 80% in detecting involved para-aortic lymph nodes.
- **E.** less than 15% of patients with positive para-aortic lymph nodes will have involved scalene lymph nodes.

198. Cancer of the cervix in pregnancy:
- **A.** occurs at an approximate rate of 1 in 2500 pregnancies.
- **B.** tends to be diagnosed later than in non-pregnant women of the same age.
- **C.** stage for stage has a worse outcome than in non-pregnant women.
- **D.** is more likely to be adenocarcinoma.
- **E.** usually presents as a result of an abnormal cervical smear.

199. Carcinoma of the vagina:
- **A.** usually occurs as a result of direct spread from an adjacent structure or by metastasis.
- **B.** when a primary, accounts for 1–2% of all genital tract malignancies in women.
- **C.** is usually either an adenocarcinoma or a melanoma.
- **D.** occurs as a primary lesion, most frequently in association with a ring pessary.
- **E.** has a better prognosis if it occurs in the lower vagina than in the upper vagina.

200. In choriocarcinoma:
- **A.** histological examination often shows pleomorphic cytotrophoblast but absence of chorionic villi.
- **B.** a third of cases present with features of distant metastatic spread.
- **C.** the antecedent pregnancy is usually a term delivery or miscarriage.
- **D.** lymph node metastases are common.
- **E.** a characteristic snowstorm pattern is seen on uterine ultrasonography.

201. Embryonal rhabdomyosarcoma (botyroid sarcoma):
- **A.** most commonly presents in children between the ages of 5 and 10 years.
- **B.** rarely arises from the vagina.
- **C.** is best managed by pelvic exenteration.
- **D.** responds to chemotherapy containing actinomycin D.
- **E.** is rarely seen in cervical polyps, the majority of which are benign in children.

202. Cancer of the cervix:

A. is confined to the cervix in over 70% of new presentations.
B. approximately 45% of patients in the UK will die from their disease.
C. laparotomy is now recommended by FIGO as part of the staging procedure.
D. intravenous pyelography (IVP) is recommended by FIGO as part of the staging procedure.
E. a third of recurrent cases will be cured by chemotherapy.

203. With regard to the histopathology of cervical cancer:

A. adenoacanthomas are tumours with malignant squamous and glandular components.
B. small cell carcinomas (squamous) have a worse prognosis than large cell carcinomas.
C. adenocarcinomas are treated similarly to squamous cancers.
D. stage for stage the prognosis for adenocarcinomas is worse than for squamous cancers.
E. large cell non-keratinizing carcinomas are associated with an overall 5-year survival rate in excess of 75%.

204. After radical hysterectomy for carcinoma of the cervix:

A. vesicovaginal fistula is more common than ureterovaginal fistula.
B. 50% of ureterovaginal fistulas will heal spontaneously within 6 months.
C. bladder atony is a significant problem in one-third of patients.
D. extensive dissection of the uterosacral ligaments may result in severe chronic constipation.
E. the single most common cause of postoperative death is pulmonary embolism.

205. In a patient who has had a laparotomy for stage IIIc epithelial ovarian cancer (EOC) with a solitary residual disease mass of 2 × 4 cm on the sigmoid colon:

A. postoperative pelvic radiotherapy is indicated.
B. reoperation and sigmoid colectomy is indicated.
C. a single alkylating agent offers the best prospect of prolonged survival.
D. a course of combination chemotherapy which includes platinum is currently considered to be the treatment of choice.
E. carboplatin would be preferable to cisplatin if the creatinine clearance is 30 ml per minute.

206. In epithelial ovarian cancer:

A. a woman who has one affected first-degree relative has a lifetime risk of 1 in 120 of developing the disease.
B. a woman with two affected first-degree relatives has a lifetime risk of up to 40% .
C. the current epidemiological data support the concept of a single autosomal dominant gene in hereditary disease.
D. hereditary disease accounts for 25% of all cases of epithelial ovarian cancer.
E. linkage to markers on chromosome 13 have been reported.

207. Serum CA125 concentration:

A. is raised in 80–85% of all epithelial ovarian cancers.
B. is less likely to be raised in mucinous than in serous tumours.
C. shows low levels of tissue expression in stage I ovarian cancer.
D. rising during treatment for ovarian cancer is a reliable indicator of poor response to therapy.
E. is increased during menstruation.

208. Uterine sarcomas:

A. are seen in approximately 0.1% of women undergoing surgery for leiomyomas.
B. have a better prognosis if they arise within a leiomyoma than if they arise diffusely within the uterus.
C. commonly present as a result of pain and a pelvic mass.
D. most frequently present as stage I (FIGO).
E. are associated with an overall 5-year survival rate of 70%.

209. Cyclophosphamide:

A. is inactive if given by mouth.
B. can be given in doses of up to 1 g/m^2.
C. may cause haemorrhagic cystitis.
D. produces a nadir in the granulocyte count on the fifth day after administration.
E. is phase specific.

210. In FIGO stage Ia ovarian cancer:

A. all patients require postoperative adjuvant chemotherapy.
B. peritoneal washings do not contain malignant cells.
C. positive para-aortic lymph nodes do not influence the staging process.
D. tumour differentiation is an independent prognostic factor.
E. conservative surgery, preserving fertility, is possible.

211. Squamous carcinoma of the vulva, T_1, N_0, M_0:

A. is equivalent to FIGO stage I.
B. includes localized tumours up to 4 cm in maximum diameter with no evidence of nodal or distant disease.
C. if lateralized, can be managed by wide local excision and ipsilateral inguinal lymphadenectomy.
D. lymphadenectomy should include the superficial and deep inguinal nodes.
E. is radiosensitive.

212. Hormone replacement therapy (HRT) is contraindicated in women with:

A. stage IIIc ovarian cancer following primary laparotomy.
B. stage Ia endometrial cancer 24 months after total abdominal hysterectomy (TAH) and bilateral salpingo-oöphorectomy (BSO).
C. stage Ib cervical cancer (squamous) 3 months after radical hysterectomy and adjuvant pelvic radiotherapy.
D. stage III endometrial cancer 6 weeks post laparotomy.
E. stage II (FIGO) vulvar cancer 3 months after wide local excision and ipsilateral (node-negative) lymphadenectomy.

213. The symptoms of epithelial ovarian cancer include:
A. abdominal distension.
B. vague gastrointestinal symptoms.
C. vaginal discharge.
D. postmenopausal bleeding.
E. abdominal pain.

214. CA125 is raised in:
A. 80% of patients with mucinous cystadenocarcinoma of the ovary.
B. some women during menstruation.
C. patients following laparoscopy.
D. pelvic inflammatory disease.
E. some patients with endometriosis.

215. The survival of patients with epithelial ovarian cancer is increased by:
A. complete removal of macroscopic disease at initial laparotomy.
B. pelvic exenteration.
C. platinum combination chemotherapy.
D. intraperitoneal cyclophosphamide.
E. performing second-look laparotomy.

216. Patients with endodermal sinus or yolk sac tumours:
A. may mimic pregnancy at presentation.
B. hardly ever require chemotherapy.
C. should have postoperative radiotherapy.
D. require monitoring with CA125.
E. require complete surgical clearance.

217. Dysgerminoma:
A. is bilateral in 10–15% of patients.
B. has a 5-year survival rate of around 90% for all stages.
C. is highly radiosensitive.
D. should have postoperative radiotherapy.
E. should have second-look laparotomy after chemotherapy to detect residual disease.

218. The following subtypes of endometrial carcinoma have a good prognosis:
- **A.** clear cell.
- **B.** undifferentiated.
- **C.** adenoacanthoma.
- **D.** serous.
- **E.** squamous.

219. The following predispose to the development of endometrial carcinoma:
- **A.** unopposed oestrogen.
- **B.** radiation.
- **C.** oral contraception.
- **D.** tamoxifen treatment.
- **E.** hereditary non-polyposis colonic cancer.

220. A laparotomy for endometrial cancer should include:
- **A.** peritoneal washings for cytology.
- **B.** total hysterectomy and bilateral salpingo-oöphorectomy.
- **C.** para-aortic lymph node biopsy.
- **D.** routine liver biopsy.
- **E.** omentectomy.

221. The following are recognized symptoms of cervical carcinoma:
- **A.** postcoital bleeding.
- **B.** offensive vaginal discharge.
- **C.** pruritus vulvae.
- **D.** postmenopausal bleeding.
- **E.** pain.

222. In the treatment of stage Ib cervical cancer, surgery:
- **A.** should consist of total abdominal hysterectomy.
- **B.** is the treatment most commonly used.
- **C.** should be used for adenocarcinoma.
- **D.** should be preceded by radiotherapy.
- **E.** is best for neuroendocrine tumours.

223. The following subtypes of human papillomavirus (HPV) are linked with invasive carcinoma of the cervix:

A. HPV 6.
B. HPV 8.
C. HPV 16.
D. HPV 18.
E. HPV 31.

224. Concerning radiotherapy for the treatment of cervical cancer:

A. the commonest complication involves the small bowel.
B. the results are improved by neoadjuvant chemotherapy.
C. the results are improved by using misonidazole as a radiosensitizer.
D. in previously irradiated patients it may be used to treat late recurrences.
E. it is the treatment most commonly used for stage 1b.

225. The following factors have a significant effect on survival in cervical cancer:

A. lymph node involvement.
B. tumour size.
C. parametrial spread.
D. depth of invasion.
E. size of lymph node metastases.

226. Vulvar cancer:

A. may present with pain.
B. is most frequently seen in the seventh decade.
C. is found more frequently in transplant patients.
D. is often seen in association with vulvar intraepithelial neoplasia (VIN) in the older woman.
E. may be metastasis from breast cancer.

227. Paget's disease of the vulva:

A. makes up 2% of all vulvar malignancies.
B. has an underlying adnexal carcinoma in 80% of cases.
C. may be associated with extragenital cancer.
D. is found most commonly in the third decade.
E. has a very poor prognosis.

228. Malignant melanoma of the vulva:
- **A.** has a better prognosis than limb melanomas.
- **B.** accounts for 5% of vulvar cancers.
- **C.** should be treated by radical vulvectomy.
- **D.** tends to occur in younger women.
- **E.** the prognosis correlates well with tumour depth.

229. Squamous cell carcinoma of the vulva:
- **A.** accounts for over 80% of primary vulvar cancers.
- **B.** may be mimicked by tuberculosis.
- **C.** should be treated by simple vulvectomy in women over 75 years of age.
- **D.** is resistant to radiotherapy.
- **E.** has a 5-year survival rate of over 30% even when the patient presents with stage 4 disease.

230. Hydatidiform mole:
- **A.** occurs once in 1200–1500 pregnancies in the West.
- **B.** may present with a small for dates uterus.
- **C.** may be complicated by shock lung after evacuation.
- **D.** has only maternal chromosomes.
- **E.** is best diagnosed by ultrasonography.

231. Risk factors for the development of malignant gestational trophoblastic neoplasia include:
- **A.** delayed postevacuation bleeding.
- **B.** pre-evacuation uterine size of greater than 20 weeks.
- **C.** gestational age.
- **D.** high initial β-hCG concentration (>100,000 iu/L).
- **E.** combined oral contraceptive use following evacuation.

232. Granulosa cell tumours:
- **A.** often behave as low-grade malignant tumours.
- **B.** often secrete oestrogen.
- **C.** are best treated by surgical removal in the first instance.
- **D.** may be macrocystic.
- **E.** may be easily diagnosed by aspiration cytology.

233. With regard to endometrial adenocarcinoma, the following are correct:
- **A.** the most common type is endometrioid.
- **B.** depth of myometrial invasion is an important prognostic factor.
- **C.** unopposed oestrogen is an important causative agent.
- **D.** the serous histological type has a good prognosis.
- **E.** the clear cell histological type has a poorer prognosis than the endometrioid type.

234. Uterine leiomyosarcoma:
- **A.** usually arises in a pre-existing benign leiomyoma.
- **B.** has similar overall 5-year survival rate to endometrial carcinoma.
- **C.** usually metastasizes via the bloodstream.
- **D.** is often associated with ovarian hyperthecosis.
- **E.** is more common in Afro-Caribbean patients.

235. In CIN-3:
- **A.** glandular acinar formations extend into the endocervical stroma.
- **B.** neoplastic cells extend into the proximal cervical glands, whereas the basal membrane remains intact.
- **C.** neoplastic cells derive from both squamous and glandular endocervical epithelium.
- **D.** there is extension of neoplastic epithelium into endocervical glands and the connective tissue.
- **E.** the diagnosis must be confirmed by biopsy.

236. Side-effects of cisplatin include:
- **A.** pulmonary fibrosis.
- **B.** haemorrhagic cystitis.
- **C.** hypocalcaemia.
- **D.** papillitis.
- **E.** alopecia.

237. An increased incidence of endometrial carcinoma is found in women with:

A. early menarche.
B. premature menopause.
C. obesity.
D. polycystic ovarian disease.
E. a history of taking the combined oral contraceptive pill.

238. Serum CA125 levels may be raised in association with:

A. epithelial ovarian cancer.
B. pregnancy.
C. endometriosis.
D. pelvic inflammatory disease.
E. renal failure.

239. With regard to minimal access surgery (MAS) in oncology:

A. laparoscopic lymphadenectomy removes as many nodes as conventional surgery.
B. extended hysterectomy, taking the parametrium, is impossible by the vaginal route.
C. laparoscopic lymphadenectomy in cervical cancer, before hysterectomy, helps stage the disease.
D. the techniques could be used to remove groin nodes in cases of vulval cancer.
E. it has a place in the prevention of ovarian cancer.

Answers

184. D

The incidence of vulvar cancer has remained much the same over the past 20 years, although there has been a reported rise in the incidence of vulvar intraepithelial neoplasia. The latter may reflect an observation effect, but a population-based survey performed in the USA suggests a real effect. The frequency with which vulvar intraepithelial neoplasia progresses to cancer is still somewhat debatable but it is unlikely to be higher than 10% of cases and probably more in the elderly and immunosuppressed. Whilst conditions such as lichen sclerosus and squamous cell hyperplasia (maturation disorders) were previously thought to be quite benign, the observation that up to one-half of cases of carcinoma may have associated maturation disorders has cast doubt on this concept. Currently the relationship is one of association and not necessarily a shared aetiology. Women with carcinoma of the vulva are at an increased risk of developing cervical carcinoma (and vice versa), this may reflect a shared aetiological agent, perhaps oncogenic human papillomavirus (HPV). Condylomata accuminata, however, are caused by non-oncogenic HPV subtypes and, whilst indicating exposure to other potential oncogens, do not in themselves become malignant.

185. BC

Small localized vulval lesions do not require removal of the whole vulva; in lateralized lesions there may often be scope for clitoral preservation which is important in sexually active women. Lateral lesions drain to the ipsilateral nodes, and the contralateral nodes are rarely or never involved unless the ipsilateral nodes are positive. Lesions involving central structures, however, may drain to both groins and, in this situation, both groins should be explored and the nodes removed. There is no evidence of increased recurrence if separate groin incisions are used for small (less than 4 cm) lesions. Superficially invasive disease (less than 1 mm invasion) is rarely associated with groin node metastasis and therefore does not warrant groin node dissection. It used to be thought that if the deep femoral nodes were involved then it was appropriate to dissect the iliac chain. This has never been shown to improve outcome and, while it may be an indication for adjuvant pelvic radiotherapy, extended node dissection is not now recommended. Age alone is not an indication to perform an inadequate operation.

186. BC

Although the subtypes 'basaloid' and 'bowenoid' are recognizable in VIN, they may be present in the same lesion and are not believed to have any prognostic value. In patients with multicentric disease there is believed to be a greater risk of progression from any of the foci (i.e. cervix, vulva, anus). While this could represent a common oncogen such as human papillomavirus (HPV), it may also reflect a disordered host response to a relatively common viral infection. The most common site for VIN is the posterior third of the inner labium minus extending to the frenulum of the fourchette. Almost two-thirds of lesions are multifocal. In non-hair-bearing skin, laser destruction to 1 mm will destroy 99% of lesions; in hair-bearing skin, destruction to a depth of 2 mm will achieve similar success. The results of treatment with 5-FU have been very disappointing, with failure rates varying between 38 and 100%.

187. AB

Cervical cancer has a wide variation in incidence. In the more developed Western countries it is relatively uncommon but in the Third World it is very prevalent. Apart from geographical variations there are also age-related differences. In the UK there has been a noticeable increase in incidence in young women. The disease spreads locoregionally and by lymphatics, the pelvic nodes being involved in about 15% of stage I cases. Despite this, staging is clinical and does not depend on a knowledge of the involvement or non-involvement of pelvic nodes. Stage IVa disease implies spread to and involvement of either the rectum or bladder. In both of these situations, exenteration may offer the chance of cure, although it is important to exclude extrapelvic disease. All tumours are potentially radiosensitive, the response is dose dependent and radioresistance implies that it is either impossible or impractical to deliver the required dose of radiation without major morbidity. There are no data supporting the concept of radioresistance in adenocarcinoma of the cervix and the current consensus is that adenocarcinomas and squamous carcinomas should be treated similarly.

188. DE

The minimum dose of radiation felt to be adequate is at least 50 Gy, although higher doses are usually employed. There has been much interest in pretreatment and or concurrent use of chemotherapy to reduce tumour volume and to radiosensitize. No clinical trial has yet established a survival advantage associated with such strategies. The propensity for lymphatic spread is well established in cervical cancer, and disease may involve the para-aortic nodes, albeit less frequently than the pelvic nodes. Despite this, it is unusual for this area to be treated unless there are good grounds for suspecting involvement. This probably reflects the increased difficulty for adequate treatment of this area and the increased morbidity associated with para-aortic irradiation. Radiation to cervical cancers involves careful calculation of the rectal dose as this is the most sensitive pelvic structure. Diarrhoea during treatment is very common and reflects the transient mild radiation enteritis. Long-term sequelae of radiation include second cancers, which may occur many years after radiation exposure.

189. C

Serum AFP levels may raised in many tumour types but is increased with any frequency only in endodermal sinus tumours. Patients with raised levels may have their chemotherapy and subsequent follow-up monitored by serial marker measurement. Increased levels reliably predate symptomatic relapse in those who were initially marker positive. Other germ cell tumours do not frequently secrete AFP although β human chorionic gonadotrophin (hCG) may be secreted by choriocarcinomas of the ovary. Stromal tumours, which include the granulosa cell tumours and arrhenoblastomas, are more likely to produce steroid hormones such as oestrogen and androgen, reflecting the function of the ovarian stroma. Epithelial tumours generally secrete CA125, although many have no clinically useful marker production.

190. CDE

Cisplatin is a useful cytotoxic agent for the treatment of epithelial ovarian cancers and is also used to treat several other malignancies. The toxicity of the drug differs from that of the other frequently used platinum compound (carboplatin). Alopecia is uncommon with cisplatin, as is myelotoxicity. Renal toxicity is, however, a problem and normal renal function is necessary before treatment. Furthermore, adequate hydration must be maintained during and for 24 hours after administration; patients are usually admitted for treatment and have a continuous saline infusion. Antiemetic drugs are virtually always prescribed as cisplatin is a powerful emetic agent. The drug is usually given in doses from 75 to 100 mg per m^2 and six to eight courses spaced 3–4 weeks apart are planned. Troublesome peripheral neuropathy, ototoxicity and deterioration in renal function are seen with increasing frequency as the total cumulative dose increases.

191. ACDE

The vulval lymphatics drain preferentially to the inguinal lymph nodes, although the frequency with which this occurs depends on the tumour type and volume. Melanomas penetrating to a depth of 10 mm have a very poor prognosis and it has not been possible to demonstrate any better disease control or indeed survival associated with lymph node dissection. Basal cell carcinomas, verrucous carcinomas and superficially invasive carcinomas have a very low incidence of lymph node metastasis and therefore groin node dissection is not usually justifiable. Frank invasive squamous cancers, however, are associated with a significant incidence of lymphatic metastases and groin node dissection is currently recommended. Recurrence of tumour in the groin is associated with a poor outcome, whereas local vulval recurrence may often be amenable to further resection.

192. AB

Most authorities would now recognize an increased incidence of disease over the past 20 years. This increase has been ascribed to an ageing population and also to the increased use of exogenous oestrogens. The median age of diagnosis for corpus cancer is 61 years and the largest number of cases is found in the 55–59-year-old age group. Five per cent are under the age of 40 years at diagnosis and between 20 and 25% are premenopausal. Most are adenocarcinomas and it is not uncommon to see metaplastic cells also. Squamous metaplasia in an adenocarcinoma is termed adenoacanthoma. This variant has a similar outcome to that of ordinary adenocarcinoma, although adenosquamous cancer (containing malignant squamous elements) has a worse outcome. Several so-called precursor lesions have been identified. These include cystic hyperplasia, adenomatous and atypical. Very few follow-up studies have been performed but two prospective series in women with an intact uterus have suggested that up to 80% of women with atypical hyperplasia will develop cancer. The risk associated with adenomatous hyperplasia is about 25%. The most recent FIGO staging (1989) recognizes three substages. Stage Ia is defined as tumour confined to the endometrium, stage Ib as that involving the inner half of the myometrium and stage Ic the outer half.

193. ADE

The most recent FIGO staging for cervical cancer now recognizes stage Ia1 as stromal invasion of no more than 3 mm with a maximum lateral spread of 7 mm. This replaces the previous definition where the maximum depth was 1 mm. The reason for this is the very low rate of nodal metastasis seen in lesions of less than 3 mm (1.3%). Stage Ia2 lesions (3–5 mm) have a higher nodal metastasis rate. Microinvasive carcinomas cannot be reliably diagnosed clinically and most usually are found as a result of investigating an abnormal cervical smear. Very few are symptomatic. It is difficult to compute the overall incidence of the condition because of the difficulties and indeed variation of pathology reporting, but stage Ia cancers overall are considered to represent about one-fifth of all invasive cervical cancers (in the Western world) and up to 7% of CIN 2 and CIN 3 (CIN, cerivcal intra-epithelial neoplasia) have been reported to contain microinvasive elements. This must be set against a background of overreporting, which some have suggested is as high as 40%. Stage Ia refers to squamous cancers only. It has not yet been possible to gain consensus on recognition of microinvasive adenocarcinomas.

194. AD

Stromal tumours account for approximately 7% of ovarian malignancies and granulosa cell tumours are the most frequently recognized stromal cancers (70%). Although many follow a slow and indolent course, sometimes over many years, they are all malignant. As with most stromal tumours, steroid hormone production is quite common, and oestrogen the most frequent. This results in up to two-thirds of patients presenting with abnormal vaginal bleeding. This is usually postmenopausal bleeding, as the average age of presentation is 52 years. Continuous unopposed excessive oestrogen results in endometrial anomalies and in one small series of 69 studied cases 22% were found to have adenocarcinoma of the endometrium, although others have reported a value of around 10%. Unlike epithelial malignancies, the majority of granulosa cell tumours present while still confined to the ovary (stage I). This statement must be qualified as the rarity of the tumour has precluded any systematic staging studies. Nevertheless in three of the largest series published, between 78% and 91% of tumours presented as stage I.

195. ABC

Survival in endometrial cancer appears to be independently related to age in that patients under the age of 59 years have an improved outcome compared with that in older patients. This may be a result of younger patients having smaller and more well-differentiated lesions, and also that the host's immune competence may be better. Stage relates closely to outcome. The prognosis for patients with stage II lesions (cervical involvement) is much worse than for those with earlier lesions. Location of the lesion within the corpus might also be significant as tumours low in the cavity might involve the cervix earlier. Tumour differentiation has long been accepted as one of the most sensitive indicators of prognosis and correlates with other factors such as degree of myometrial penetration and lymph node metastasis. Obesity, diabetes mellitus and hypertension are classically related to increased risk of endometrial cancer, although they could be associated phenomena seen with increasing frequency in an ageing female population. They in themselves do not directly affect outcome but might prejudice the ability to deliver effective treatment.

196. BD

Colposcopy alone probably has a 70% accuracy in suspecting microinvasive disease, which like all epithelial abnormalities requires a biopsy to confirm the diagnosis. In between one-third and one-half of cases of microinvasion, colposcopy is unsatisfactory because the squamocolumnar junction (SCJ) is sited within the endocervical canal. This may reflect the age group of the patients concerned and underlines the importance of an excisional procedure (cone biopsy) if the SCJ cannot be fully visualized. Acetowhite epithelium and mosaicism may well be present in cases of invasive disease but are usually associated with underlying CIN and not invasion. They are seen frequently enough in patients with abnormal cervical smears as not to be suggestive of invasion. Leucoplakia, or surface hyperkeratosis, might mask underlying features of invasion but in itself is not suggestive of invasion. Indeed leucoplakia is not infrequently seen in cases of human papillomavirus infection. Atypical vessels and irregularity of the surface contour are considered to indicate an underlying invasive process and, if either of these features is recognized, a large excisional biopsy should be performed to exclude this possibility.

197. ACDE

Whilst one must accept that data pertaining to node positivity with stage suffer from certain inaccuracies, both in staging and in node sampling error, large pooled series of data have been used to approximate node positivity. These data, based on over 1700 patients, showed that the pelvic node positivity rate for stage Ib cancers was 19.8%. In the same series there were 23 cases of stage IVa disease and the pelvic node positivity rate was 55%. Nodal spread from the pelvic to the para-aortic and thence to the scalene is a well recognized phenomenon. Those who have clinical IIb disease (again from pooled data and relating to 602 cases of stage IIb) have 19.8% involvement of the para-aortic nodes. When scalene nodes have been sampled, 11 of 83 patients with positive para-aortic node disease were found to have disease in the scalene nodes (13%). Figures such as these justify continued attempts to find useful, parenteral, adjuvant therapies for cervical cancer.

198. AB

Cancer of the cervix is uncommon in pregnancy, the average incidence in large centres being 1 in 2500. Abnormal smears and preinvasive disease are much more common (CIN 3 reported as 1 in 750 pregnancies and approximately 10–15 abnormal smears reported per 1000 pregnancies). Unfortunately the diagnosis is often delayed with the youth of the patient, the accompanying pregnancy making clinicians somewhat reluctant to investigate at the first sign of abnormal bleeding. All cases of excessive discharge or vaginal bleeding during pregnancy should be assessed at least by speculum examination. The lateness of diagnosis has led to a consensus in the literature that cancer of the cervix diagnosed in the latter part of pregnancy or in the immediate puerperium has a grave prognosis. Stage for stage, however, the outcome is no different from that in the non-pregnant state. There would appear to be a high degree of squamous differentiation in pregnancy, although the overall pattern of histological findings does not differ from that seen in non-pregnant women. Most cases of cervical cancer are symptomatic in pregnancy and vaginal bleeding is the most common symptom. Taking smears during pregnancy is now discouraged unless none has been taken within the previous 5 years. Cytology screening is best conducted outside pregnancy as the quality of smears is better. Finally, in countries that operate a structured cytology screening programme, there are few if any indications to take *ad hoc* smears outwith the programme.

199. AB

Carcinoma of the vagina is very uncommon and most of the tumours found in the vagina occur as a result of spread from the cervix, vulva, rectum, bladder or endometrium. In its primary form it accounts for only 1–2% of all genital tract cancers. Most carcinomas are squamous (>90%) developing in women with a mean age of 60 years. Adenocarcinoma accounts for between 4 and 5% and, although there is a recognized association between clear cell adenocarcinoma and diethylstilboestrol exposure in utero, some authorities now recognize an increase in the incidence of adenocarcinoma that is unrelated to such exposure. No single aetiological agent has been identified. Historically it has been taught that squamous cancer arises in procidentias and ring pessary ulcers. However, four relatively large series (published between 1971 and 1983) with a total of 276 cases related either procidentia or a pessary as the cause in only 18 cases. The most common site for vaginal cancer is the posterior upper third of the vagina, followed by the anterior lower third. It has been noted that the prospect for cure is better when lesions are confined to the upper vagina. This may be because of similarities to cervical cancer and ease of treatment, and also because the upper vagina is more distensible than the lower vagina so that infiltration of subepithelial tissues occurs later.

200. ABC

The histology of choriocarcinoma is characterized by pleomorphic cytotrophoblast surrounded by some syncytium with extensive areas of haemorrhage. Chorionic villi are not seen. The majority of patients present within 1 year of an apparently normal pregnancy or non-molar miscarriage; however, choriocarcinoma is much more likely to occur following a hydatidiform mole (1500 times more likely than after a normal pregnancy), although such events are much less common than normal pregnancies. Vaginal bleeding with or without discharge is the most common symptom, although one-third of cases present as a result of symptoms arising from distant metastases, pulmonary, cerebral and hepatic deposits being the most frequent. Lymph node and bone metastases are rare and, if present, should suggest a histological review as the pathology may not be choriocarcinoma. Ultrasonography is useful in determining uterine size and monitoring response to therapy, although estimation of hCG activity is the most reliable monitor of response. The characteristic 'snowstorm' pattern seen with hydatidiform moles is not seen with choriocarcinoma.

201. D

Embryonal rhabdomyosarcoma is a highly malignant lesion most commonly seen in the very young (2 years of age or less). In the youngest children the tumour usually originates in the lower vagina, in older ones the upper vagina and cervix, although there are exceptions to this rule. Simple benign polyps of the vagina and cervix are extremely unusual in children and any polypoid structure in the lower genital tract in children should be treated with suspicion and always biopsied. The treatment of this tumour has changed with the advent of effective multiple-agent chemotherapy. Exenterative surgery is now used only in those not responding or only partially responding to chemotherapy (which usually contains actinomycin D). Radiotherapy is not frequently employed because of the long-term effects on pelvic bone development.

202. BD

Despite the fact that a screening programme is now in place, the most recent epidemiological data indicate that almost one-half of new presentations are advanced in that the disease has spread beyond the confines of the cervix at the time of presentation. This, not surprisingly, results in an overall 5-year survival rate somewhat lower than might be expected. In the UK approximately 45% of patients will die within 5 years. Cervical cancer is well recognized as spreading both locally and by the local lymphatics. Lymph node status is not yet recognized as part of staging, which remains a clinical exercise and does not require exploratory laparotomy, although many centres are increasingly using both laparotomy and less invasive investigative techniques in an attempt to assess nodal involvement. Ureteric obstruction remains a major prognostic variable in cervical cancer and the staging committee of FIGO recommends IVP as a part of staging. Five per cent of clinical stage Ib cancers will be upstaged as a result of IVP investigations. The management of relapsed disease remains a major problem. In patients treated initially by surgery, radiotherapy is the treatment of first choice for local relapse, and exenterative surgery may salvage up to 50% of local central pelvic relapses after primary radiotherapy. In those where neither treatment modality is feasible, chemotherapy offers a good chance of response, but few if any patients maintain this response and less than 5% can expect any long-term remission.

203. BCE

Cervical cancers are most commonly squamous but malignant change in the glandular epithelium of the endocervix also occurs. If both components show malignant features the tumour is termed an adenosquamous tumour. Adenoacanthoma applies to the situation when the tumour is an adenocarcinoma but benign squamous metaplasia is seen (as is the case for endometrial carcinoma). Several types of squamous differentiation are seen. Small cell carcinoma generally has a worse prognosis than the large cell variety and this relates to the degree of differentiation. The more like normal squamous epithelium, the better the prognosis, so that large cell non-keratinizing carcinomas are generally regarded as the most 'normally differentiated' and associated with the best outcome. Despite the recognized association between histological findings and behaviour of the tumour, this has not yet resulted in altered treatment strategies, and the two largest subgroups (adenocarcinoma and squamous cancer) are managed similarly. Furthermore, stage for stage (and, perhaps more accurately, volume for volume), it has not been possible to demonstrate reliably that adenocarcinoma has a worse prognosis.

204. BDE

Over the past two decades improvements in preoperative and postoperative care, along with improvements in surgical technique, have greatly reduced the morbidity associated with radical hysterectomy. A high incidence of ureterovaginal fistula was considered to be one of the major problems. This occurs much less frequently now, with most modern series quoting less than 2%. This is still more common than vesicovaginal fistula, which is quoted as rare and which usually heals spontaneously. Some 50% of ureterovaginal fistulas will close spontaneously within 6 months and any attempt at repair should be delayed for this length of time to allow for spontaneous healing and also for any inflammatory reaction to subside, as this will facilitate further surgical correction. Bladder atony was also considered to be a significant problem in the past, but no longer. Similarly, disturbance of bowel function (mainly severe constipation) can occur but is unusual as extensive dissection of the uterosacral ligaments (deep and medial, particularly) is no longer considered to be necessary in the majority of patients selected for primary surgical treatment. Operative mortality has declined steadily as to almost approach zero. The most likely cause of postoperative death is now pulmonary embolism. Careful attention to thromboprophylaxis can minimize this event.

205. DE

The majority of patients with advanced disease will have residual tumour at the conclusion of primary laparotomy. Patients who achieve maximal clearance (i.e. no residual disease) have a better prognosis but, as yet, those who achieve this state as a result of further debulking have not been shown to enjoy the same survival advantage. Interval or secondary debulking surgery cannot therefore be recommended as standard practice and should be reserved for controlled trials. There are currently few, if any, indications for pelvic radiotherapy in ovarian cancer. Essentially it is regarded as a disseminated disease, so localized therapy is of little use in a curative setting. There will, however, be occasions where palliation might be achieved via this route. Postoperative treatment in EOC relies almost entirely on chemotherapy. Initially this was based on alkylating agents such as cyclophosphamide and melphalan. In the past 15 years the emphasis has shifted to the use of platinum-based chemotherapy. This generates both higher response rates and improved median survival compared with alkylating agents alone. Cisplatinum is, however, nephrotoxic and where there is evidence of renal compromise, carboplatin (a platinum analogue with a different toxicity profile but similar efficacy) is preferred.

206. BC

Data from the Office of Population Censuses and Surveys (OPCS) in the UK have suggested that the lifetime risk of developing epithelial ovarian cancer in a woman who has one affected first-degree female relative is approximately 1 in 40 or about three times the risk in the general population. This risk increases to a lifetime risk of 30–40% in women who have two affected first-degree relatives. These epidemiological data are highly suggestive, although not confirmatory, of a single autosomal gene effect. This does not preclude the possibility of more than one predisposing gene and the situation can be resolved only by means of genetic linkage studies. Chromosome 17 has been implicated on the basis of such genetic linkage studies (comparing the frequency of the observed phenotypes with known genetic markers on the chromosome in question). Despite the large amount of interest in the possible genetic predisposition to ovarian cancer, currently less than 5% of all cases are considered to be hereditary.

207. ABDE

CA125 is an antigenic determinant on a high molecular weight glycoprotein expressed by epithelial ovarian tumours and other tissues of Müllerian origin. Its level is increased above the normal value (35 units/ml) before operation in 80–85% of women with EOC. Although, initially, mucinous tumours were considered to be CA125 negative, several reports have now suggested an increase in up to 66% of mucinous cystadenocarcinomas. Levels are, however, less frequently raised in this subtype of epithelial tumours. Much interest has been shown in trying to utilize this tumour marker as part of a screening programme. On its own, it is increased in only 50% of stage I tumours. This is not because of poor tissue expression but more likely as a result of factors other than synthesis; stage I cancers are seen to express the antigen in up to 90% of cases. The clinical utility of the markers currently lies in its ability to monitor therapy. Rapidly falling levels generally indicate a good response to treatment, whereas persistently high or rising levels indicate a poor outcome and may well form the basis of discontinuing or changing treatment. The marker is non-specific. Pregnancy and menstruation are associated with increased levels of the marker, although these are generally far less marked than in cancer. Similarly, benign conditions such as endometriosis and pelvic sepsis may cause an increase in the serum concentration.

208. ABD

Uterine sarcomas are rare with a reported incidence of 0.67 per 100,000 women aged 20 years and older. One large survey has suggested that 0.13% of all fibroids removed will contain sarcoma. This figure, however, is very variable as it will depend, to some extent, on the indications used to undertake surgery for 'benign' pelvic masses. It is also highly dependent on the criteria used to diagnose leiomyosarcoma. Sarcomas arising within a fibroid appear to have a better prognosis than those that occur diffusely within the uterus although, once again, the rarity of such tumours renders appropriate multivariate analysis of prognostic factors difficult and such data are usually the result of individual series. Abnormal vaginal bleeding accounts for two-thirds of all presentations, pain being a feature of presentation in about 38% of patients. Stage I disease, or disease confined to the uterine fundus, is the most common (63%) and most survivors will be found within this group with very localized disease. Even in those with apparent stage I disease, the 5-year survival rate is poor and estimated at no higher than 50%. Prognosis appears to be closely related to mitotic count, any case with more than 10 mitoses per 10 high power fields being associated with a poor outcome (only 3 of 36 survivors in one series). If all cases are considered, the 5-year survival rate falls to 40%.

209. BC

Cyclophosphamide is frequently used in the treatment of gynaecological malignancies and most often in ovarian cancer. It is an alkylating agent and, like other alkylating agents, is not phase specific. This means it can affect cell division at a variety of sites; thus the activity and toxicity of these agents are very variable. Cyclophosphamide can be given by mouth and used to be instilled intraperitoneally after surgery. As the drug becomes active only after passage through the liver, peritoneal administration is now considered inappropriate. Most alkylating agents have a degree of marrow toxicity (cisplatin has very little) and serial measurement of the white cell count (WCC) is important in patients treated with cyclophosphamide. Extremely low white counts are associated with sepsis and these infections require active intervention and patient support until the count has recovered. Following treatment with cyclophosphamide (400–1000 mg/m^2 intravenously), the nadir in WCC occurs between 8 and 14 days, with recovery at 18–25 days. The drug has a relatively long half-life and is excreted via the kidney. High levels in the urine may result in haemorrhagic cystitis.

210. BDE

Stage Ia (FIGO) ovarian cancer is defined as malignant change confined to an ovary and not breaching the ovarian capsule.

A survival rate in excess of 80% at 5 years is expected in properly staged cases. Staging involves peritoneal lavage in the absence of ascites; the presence of malignant cells means that the stage would be Ic. Rupture of the cyst at the time of surgery also requires the case to be upstaged. Sampling of the retroperitoneal nodes is also included in the operative staging process and any evidence of nodal disease will result in upstaging to stage III. Despite the high success rate of surgery alone, a proportion of patients will relapse. Prognostic factors of value in predicting relapse of stage I cases are substage (Ic versus Ia) and tumour differentiation. Adjuvant chemotherapy is not of proven value but trials addressing this issue would normally recognize candidates for chemotherapy from within the poorly differentiated tumours. Accurate staging procedures do not require removal of the uterus and both ovaries. It is important, however, to take representative biopsies from the remaining ovary.

211. ACDE

Both staging systems (TNM and FIGO) are used in describing spread of vulvar cancer. T_1 lesions are those confined to the vulva and less than 2 cm in diameter; this corresponds to FIGO stage I lesions. Although the suspicion of groin node metastasis is included in the TNM classification, it is notoriously unreliable with almost 50% of cases with non-suspicious nodes having at least microscopic metastases. The outcome of vulval cancer is related directly to nodal status. The 5-year survival rate in node-negative cases is over 80% whereas positivity confers a rate of 50% or less. For this reason, great emphasis is placed on the likelihood of node positivity. Lateralized lesions less than 4 cm in diameter rarely if ever involve the contralateral nodes if the ipsilateral nodes are negative, and should therefore be managed initially by ipsilateral lymphadenectomy, only proceeding to a contralateral dissection if the ipsilateral nodes are positive. Similar observations have been made with regard to nodal depth. If the superficial inguinal nodes are negative, the deep nodes rarely if ever harbour metastases. Despite this, the current consensus is to remove the superficial and deep nodes at the same time, largely because a second dissection in the groin is technically more difficult and, as yet, frozen section cannot reliably rule out metastases in the total superficial dissection. There may be scope, however, to consider radiotherapy to the deep nodes if the superficial nodes are found to be positive, as the tumour is not resistant to radiotherapy and modern radiotherapeutic techniques have been shown to be of value in treating some of these cancers.

212. D

HRT can result in major improvements in the quality of life. In the care of patients with cancer, adversely affecting prognosis must always be balanced against improvements in the quality of life. The only information pertaining to the potential for HRT to affect prognosis adversely is in endometrial cancer, which in a proportion of cases is an oestrogen-dependent tumour. For this reason, patients who have ovarian, cervical or vulval tumours should not be denied HRT if required for quality-of-life reasons. Furthermore, there are also arguments for supporting the use of HRT in selected cases of endometrial cancer where the risk of relapse is low and where the benefits may be high.

213. ABDE

Although ovarian cancer is known as the 'silent killer', it gives rise to a number of symptoms, especially in patients with advanced disease. Stage I tumours may present with pain due to torsion, rupture, haemorrhage or infection. Advanced disease may present with pain (50.8%), abdominal swelling (49.5%), anorexia (21.6%), nausea and vomiting (21.6%), weight loss (17.5%), vaginal bleeding (17.1%), frequency (16.4%), change in bowel habit and malaise.

214. BCDE

OC125 is a murine monoclonal antibody that was first raised by R.C. Bast and R.C. Knapp. The determinant to which OC125 binds has been designated CA125. This antigen is expressed by coelomic epithelium and amnion during fetal development. It is not associated with normal ovarian tissue in either the fetus or the adult. It is detected in 80% of non-mucinous epithelial ovarian cancers. Raised levels may be found in other gynaecological cancers arising from coelomic epithelial derivatives (including fallopian tube, endometrium and endocervix). CA125 concentration is also raised in the majority of pancreatic cancers and in a minority of patients with breast, lung and colonic cancers. As a result, it is of no help in locating the origin of peritoneal carcinomatosis from an unknown primary. Raised levels are found in conditions and diseases that irritate the peritoneum such as acute pancreatitis, peritonitis, pelvic inflammatory disease and endometriosis. Its level is also increased during the first trimester of normal pregnancy and occasionally during menstruation. Despite the development of other markers such as CA19-9, CA125 remains the most useful marker used in the management of epithelial ovarian cancer. Its use in any screening programme for ovarian cancer is limited by the fact that its level is increased in approximately 10% of apparently healthy women.

215. AC

The 5-year survival rate for patients with complete macroscopic clearance of tumour at initial laparotomy is around 70%, compared with 20–30% for those with macroscopic residual disease. Whether the difference is due to surgery or to a difference in the biology of the disease is not known. There is no evidence that more radical surgery, such as exenteration, is of any benefit in advanced disease. Meta-analysis has shown a slight advantage for platinum-containing combination chemotherapy against single agents including cisplatinum. Cyclophosphamide needs to be activated by the liver; therefore, it is of no use given intraperitoneally. Second-look laparotomy is an operation performed at the completion of first-line chemotherapy. The idea was that it would confer a survival advantage either by detecting residual disease early or by removing any residual disease. Neither of these theoretical advantages has been realized, probably because of the poor results of second-line chemotherapy. At present second-look laparotomy has no part to play in the management of epithelial ovarian cancer and should be performed only in the context of a study.

216. A

Endodermal sinus tumours produce β-hCG and α-fetoprotein. The median age at presentation is 19 years, which explains why the wrong diagnosis of pregnancy is made occasionally. Before the introduction of combination chemotherapy, even stage I disease had an appalling prognosis with an 80% mortality rate. With modern combination chemotherapy (e.g. bleomycin, cisplatin and vinblastine or etoposide) the complete response rate is in excess of 80% and the overall cure rate exceeds 70%. These tumours are so chemosensitive that cytoreductive surgery is unnecessary and surgery is needed only to obtain a histological diagnosis.

217. ABC

Although dysgerminomas are highly radiosensitive, they are also highly chemosensitive. As a result postoperative radiotherapy is no longer used. Recurrences after surgery are treated by chemotherapy using combinations such as cisplatin, bleomycin and vinblastine. Recently etoposide has been used in place of vinblastine. Patients with advanced disease now have their fertility conserved by conservative surgery and chemotherapy. This is extremely important in the management of a disease that is usually found in girls or young women. Second-look laparotomy is no longer used to detect residual disease, because almost all residual masses following chemotherapy have been found to consist of fibrous tissue only.

218. C

The prognosis of patients with endometrial cancer is determined by the stage of disease, lymph node status, depth of myometrial invasion, grade of differentiation and histological subtype. Adenoacanthomas have benign squamous metaplasia and do not differ in prognosis from the usual adenocarcinoma. The other subtypes have a poorer prognosis, especially serous and clear cell types.

219. ABDE

A number of factors are known to predispose to the development of endometrial carcinoma including obesity, unopposed oestrogen, radiation and tamoxifen. Although it is generally accepted that tamoxifen induces certain changes (including cancer) in the endometrium, it must be borne in mind that its benefits in the treatment of breast cancer outweigh any ill effects it may have on the endometrium. Women from families that suffer from hereditary non-polyposis colonic cancer (HNPCC) have a 30% chance of developing endometrial cancer in their lifetime and should be monitored for this.

220. ABC

Endometrial cancer is probably the least well staged of all gynaecological cancers. It is seldom referred to a gynaecological oncology unit, probably because most gynaecologists erroneously believe that it has a better prognosis than cervical or ovarian cancer. The present FIGO staging takes account of histological findings, i.e. it is now surgically staged:

Stage Ia	Tumour limited to endometrium
Stage Ib	Invasion to less than one-half the myometrium
Stage Ic	Invasion to more than one-half the myometrium
Stage IIa	Endocervical glandular involvement only
Stage IIb	Cervical stromal invasion
Stage IIIa	Tumour invades serosa and/or adnexa, and/or positive peritoneal cytology
Stage IIIb	Vaginal metastases
Stage IIIc	Metastases to pelvic and/or para-aortic lymph nodes
Stage IVa	Tumour invasion of bladder and/or bowel mucosa
Stage IVb	Distant metastases including intra-abdominal organs and/or inguinal lymph nodes.

221. ABDE

Patients with cervical cancer usually present with some form of vaginal bleeding or discharge. The friable tumour epithelium often gives rise to postcoital or intermenstrual bleeding, or postmenopausal bleeding if the patient has reached the menopause. An offensive vaginal discharge is often present due either to the presence of altered blood or to the presence of infected necrotic tumour. Pain is uncommon and is almost always associated with advanced disease.

222. C

Surgery for stage Ib cervical cancer should consist of a Wertheim or radical hysterectomy. Although it should be used for most fit patients with stage Ib disease, radiotherapy remains the most commonly used modality of treatment even in developed countries. There appears to be no difference in the survival of patients with stage Ib disease treated with surgery or radiotherapy, except in those with adenocarcinoma or adenosquamous carcinoma, in whom there is evidence in favour of surgery. Neuroendocrine and small cell undifferentiated tumours have an appalling prognosis uninfluenced by the modality of treatment.

223. CDE

HPV 6 and 8 are associated with CIN whereas HPV 16, 18 and 31 are associated with cervical cancer.

224. DE

Although small bowel is easily damaged by radiation, the most common radiotherapy injuries involve the bladder or rectum. There is no evidence that either neoadjuvant chemotherapy or misonidazole improves the results of radiotherapy. A number of studies have now shown that further radiotherapy can be given safely if recurrence occurs 10 years or more following irradiation for cervical cancer.

225. ABCDE

Lymph node involvement is the most important factor in survival. Negative lymph nodes indicate a 5-year survival rate of around 90%, whereas the rate in patients with positive nodes ranges from 20 to 60%. The 5-year survival rate for patients with macroscopic lymph node disease is 54% compared with 82.5% for those with tumour emboli only.

Patients with lesions smaller than 2 cm have a 5-year-survival rate of around 90%. This is reduced to 60% for those with tumours above 2 cm and to 40% for those above 4 cm. The 5-year survival rate is around 90% for patients with negative parametria, 75% for those with microscopic involvement and 50% when both the parametrium and pelvic lymph nodes are involved. Depth of invasion under 1.5 cm is associated with a 90% 5-year survival rate, compared with 63–70% when invasion is deeper.

226. ABCE

One-third of patients with vulvar carcinoma present with pain; it is the third most common symptom after irritation and the discovery of a lump. Vulvar carcinoma is most frequently seen in the seventh decade of life, which is why these patients often have significant medical problems. A 100-fold increase in the incidence of cancer of the vulva and anus is seen in transplant patients when compared with the normal population. In the older woman vulvar carcinoma is most often seen in association with lichen sclerosus; the association of vulvar cancer and VIN is found in younger women. The vulva is not an uncommon site for metastases, particularly from the cervix, vagina, ovary, gastrointestinal tract, renal tract and even from such distant sites as the breast and thyroid.

227. ACE

Unlike Paget's disease of the breast, only one-fifth of cases have an underlying carcinoma of adnexal structures. Paget's disease has been found in association with extragenital cancer in up to 40% in some series. The disease is most commonly found in middle-aged or elderly women. The prognosis is excellent except when there is dermal invasion or an underlying adnexal carcinoma.

228. BE

Malignant melanomas of the vulva account for 5% of primary vulvar cancers. They tend to occur in older women with a mean age of over 60 years in most large series. The prognosis is worse than for melanomas of the limbs and correlates well with depth of tumour. Breslow's classification appears to be better for predicting prognosis than Clark's levels. Tumour depth of up to 0.76 mm has an excellent prognosis and should be treated by wide excision alone. Tumours of up to 1.5 mm have an intermediate prognosis and may benefit from groin node dissection. Radical vulvectomy is still carried out for this group in some centres. Tumours greater than 1.5 mm have a poor prognosis and should be treated by wide excision as radical vulvectomy does not improve survival.

229. ABE

Benign conditions such as lymphogranuloma inguinale and tuberculosis may mimic squamous cell carcinoma of the vulva, which is why all suspicious vulvar lesions should be biopsied before planning treatment. Recurrence in the groin lymph nodes is almost always fatal, whereas local recurrence is more easily salvaged. This is why simple vulvectomy is the wrong treatment for these tumours. Although surgery remains the more effective treatment, vulvar carcinomas are radiosensitive and chemosensitive. Radiotherapy has been shown to be effective in reducing the need for exenterative surgery in most cases of advanced vulvar carcinoma.

230. ABCE

Although half the patients with hydatidiform mole present with a uterus too large for dates, 20% present with a uterus that is small for dates. One of the most important of complications following evacuation of a hydatidiform mole is the postevacuation pulmonary insufficiency syndrome, or shock lung. The aetiology is uncertain but may be caused by deportation of molar tissue through venous sinuses to the lung. Most complete moles have two haploid sets of chromosomes, 46,XX, both of which are paternally derived, whereas partial moles are most often triploid with a contribution from both parents. The appearance of a hydatidiform mole on ultrasonography is diagnostic and no other test is required for diagnosis even though β-hCG and other forms of imaging may be helpful in subsequent management.

231. ABD

Risk factors for the development of malignant gestational trophoblastic neoplasia include delayed postevacuation bleeding, theca lutein cysts, uterus larger than 20 weeks' size before evacuation, previous hydatidiform mole, pulmonary insufficiency syndrome, advanced maternal age and initial β-hCG level greater than 100,000 iu/L.

Studies have shown no increased risk of malignant change in using the oral contraceptive pill following evacuation. Recently, it has even been suggested that it might be advantageous to use oral contraception after molar pregnancy.

232. ABCD

Accurate diagnosis of granulosa cell and all other sex cord-stromal tumours of the ovary is by surgical removal and histological examination. Granulosa cell tumours are typically oestrogen secreting and may lead to coexistent endometrial hyperplasia and carcinoma. Approximately half of the cases have large cysts. The 10-year survival rate varies from 60 to 90%. Before puberty and in young adults a variant type occurs, known as a juvenile granulosa cell tumour. This tumour behaves in a benign fashion in the majority of low stage cases but, when clinically malignant, progression is more rapid than for the 'adult' type.

233. ABCE

The commonest type of endometrial adenocarcinoma (the endometrioid type) is associated with unopposed oestrogenic stimulation and is often coexistent with or follows on from atypical endometrial hyperplasia. Grade I tumours generally have a favourable prognosis with a 5-year survival rate of more than 75% (all stages). Outcome is dependent on stage, depth of myometrial invasion, grade and several other factors. Serous and clear cell carcinomas of the endometrium have a considerably poorer prognosis than endometrioid, and metastasize early. They tend to occur in the elderly and do not show the same close association with oestrogenic stimulation.

234. C

Most uterine leiomyosarcomas arise *de novo*. Some 50–75% are solitary masses, and are poorly defined with necrosis and haemorrhage evident. They metastasize early via the bloodstream and the overall 5-year survival rate is only 15–25%. They are not associated with race, gravidity or parity.

235. BE

CIN-3 frequently involves the endocervical glands, and these processes can extend quite deeply into the cervical stroma. Some form of crypt involvement is likely to be found in over 80% of cases of CIN-3, and will generally be between 1 and 6 mm deep. The abnormality is confined strictly to the squamous component; there is no concomitant endocervical cellular abnormality.

236. CD

Cisplatin (alone or in combination with other cytotoxic drugs) is used in the treatment of stage III and IV epithelial ovarian cancer. Side-effects include severe nausea and vomiting, ototoxicity, myelosuppression (reaching a nadir at 3 weeks), renal failure, diarrhoea, hypomagnesaemia and hypocalcaemia (both rarely symptomatic), neuropathy, fits and papillitis.

237. CD

It has been long well recognized that oestrogens, unopposed by progestogens, lead to an increased incidence of endometrial carcinoma. This was originally (in the 1950s) suggested from the reports of a higher incidence in postmenopausal women with oestrogen-secreting ovarian tumours, and later on (in the 1970s) in women taking unopposed oestrogen hormone replacement therapy. Other conditions that lead to increased oestrogen levels and are associated with an increased incidence of endometrial carcinoma include obesity, anovulatory infertility, polycystic ovarian disease and late age of menopause. Early menarche and premature menopause have no effect on the incidence of endometrial carcinoma. Use of the combined oral contraceptive pill significantly reduces the risk of endometrial carcinoma.

238. ABCDE

CA125 is a high molecular weight glycoprotein expressed by cells derived from the embryonal coelomic epithelium and Müllerian duct. Benign and malignant pathologies affecting tissues with these embryological origins have been associated with increased CA125 expression. Over 80% of patients with epithelial ovarian cancer have increased serum levels of CA125 (>35 units/ml). However, when analysed by stage of disease, there is a skewed distribution, with raised levels in 90% of women with stage II, III and IV disease, but in only 50% of women with stage I ovarian cancer. This is rather disappointing because it is in women with early stage disease who would ideally be detected in any screening programme. Other conditions in which raised CA125 levels have been observed include pregnancy, endometriosis, pelvic inflammatory disease, adenomyosis, pancreatitis, chronic alcoholic hepatitis and renal failure. Among healthy blood donors, the levels were increased in 1% of women.

239. DE

MAS is being used increasingly in oncological procedures, but, as yet, with no published evidence that the purported immediate reduction in mortality rate is not accompanied by compromise with regard to long-term survival. Laparoscopic external iliac and obturator lymphadenectomy for cervical cancer relies on avulsion of tissue. This may be expected to cause more bleeding than painstaking conventional surgery, but this disadvantage is offset by the advantages of the minimal access technique. Results on long-term morbidity and cure rates are awaited. Early studies show a reduced number of nodes collected by MAS, but this may be a learning curve effect. Lymph node status is not part of cervical cancer staging, although it radically affects prognosis. MAS removal of pelvic nodes has allowed the resurgence of the vaginal equivalent of Wertheim's hysterectomy, described by Shauter. Removal of groin nodes in vulval cancer using MAS techniques has now been described. Laparoscopic oöphorectomy has a place in the prevention of cancer in women positive for the Lynch genetic predisposition.

4

Reproductive Medicine

Questions

240. A 20-year-old normal-looking woman complaining of secondary amenorrhoea and hot flushes was found to have raised follicle-stimulating hormone (FSH) and leutinizing hormone (LH) levels. The differential diagnosis includes the following:

A. polyglandular autoimmune endocrine failure.
B. an abnormality of the X chromosome.
C. galactosaemia.
D. Kallmann's syndrome.
E. Laurence-Moon-Biedl syndrome.

241. Premature menopause is associated with:

A. hot flushes in approximately 80% of patients.
B. galactosaemia.
C. mumps.
D. autoimmune disease.
E. high incidence of miscarriage if treated with ovum donation.

242. A low level of sex hormone-binding globulin (SHBG) is:

A. a predictor of the development of type II diabetes mellitus.
B. associated with increased bodyweight.
C. associated with low circulating insulin levels.
D. caused by hyperthyroidism.
E. caused by progestogens.

243. Hyperprolactinaemia:

A. is a recognized feature of hyperthyroidism.
B. is a side-effect of metoclopramide therapy.
C. is found in 75–80% of patients with acromegaly.
D. can be treated medically with dopamine agonists.
E. when considering pituitary pathologies is invariably due to a prolactin-secreting microadenoma.

244. Polycystic ovary syndrome:

A. as defined morphologically by ovarian ultrasonography affects 20% of all premenopausal women.
B. is characterized by increased sensitivity to insulin.
C. is the commonest cause of anovulatory infertility.
D. is associated with a negative progesterone challenge test.
E. commonly causes hyperprolactinaemia.

245. Follicle-stimulating hormone (FSH):

A. stimulates spermatogenesis from the Leydig cells of the testis.
B. level is raised in patients receiving long-term gonadotrophin-releasing hormone agonists.
C. is under negative feedback control from oestrogens and inhibin.
D. level is increased in most adult women with Turner's syndrome.
E. is suppressed in patients with Cushing's disease.

246. In patients with hirsutism:

A. circulating dehydroepiandrosterone sulphate (DHAS) is raised in the majority of cases.
B. circulating testosterone concentration is usually increased.
C. a follicular phase basal 17-hydroxyprogesterone level of less than 5 nmol/l excludes late-onset 21-hydroxylase deficiency.
D. ovarian and adrenal tumours should be excluded in patients with cliteromegaly.
E. cyproheptadine is an effective treatment.

247. Hypogonadism is a feature of:
- **A.** Kallmann's syndrome.
- **B.** Turner's syndrome.
- **C.** liver cirrhosis.
- **D.** haemochromatosis.
- **E.** Prader-Willi syndrome.

248. Precocious puberty:
- **A.** is a feature of the McCune-Albright syndrome.
- **B.** is defined as the appearance of secondary sexual development in males before the age of 12 years.
- **C.** if incomplete, should be treated with gonadotrophin-releasing hormone agonists.
- **D.** may be caused by primary hypothyroidism.
- **E.** may be caused by 21-hydroxylase deficiency.

249. During human pregnancy:
- **A.** the corpus luteum regresses within 7 days of implantation.
- **B.** progesterone is required for maintenance of the conceptus during the first 6 weeks.
- **C.** maternal cortisol values rise threefold across pregnancy, principally owing to an increase in maternal corticosteroid-binding globulin levels.
- **D.** the maternal ovary is the principal source of maternal oestrogen during the second and third trimesters.
- **E.** impaired fetal growth is associated with hypertension in later adult life.

250. Sex hormone-binding globulin (SHBG):
- **A.** in women binds approximately 25% of circulating testosterone
- **B.** concentration is increased in states of hyperandrogenism.
- **C.** concentration is raised in hypothyroidism.
- **D.** binds to 50% of circulating progesterone.
- **E.** levels are increased in patients taking the combined oral contraceptive pill.

251. Recognized causes of amenorrhoea include:
- **A.** Cushing's syndrome.
- **B.** androgen insensitivity syndromes.
- **C.** galactosaemia.
- **D.** 21-hydroxylase deficiency.
- **E.** craniopharyngioma.

252. Clomiphene citrate:
- **A.** increases pituitary gonadotrophin secretion.
- **B.** is effective in patients with premature ovarian failure.
- **C.** can cause hot flushing.
- **D.** can cause hirsutism.
- **E.** is associated with a multiple pregnancy rate of approximately 25%.

253. Recognized indications for in vitro fertilization (IVF) treatment include:
- **A.** tubal disease.
- **B.** endometriosis.
- **C.** unexplained infertility.
- **D.** oligospermia.
- **E.** premature ovarian failure.

254. In the UK the average success rates for IVF, using the woman's own eggs, are:
- **A.** approximately 25% live births per cycle started, overall.
- **B.** principally dependent on the female indication for treatment.
- **C.** principally dependent on the age of the woman.
- **D.** principally dependent on the past obstetric history of the woman.
- **E.** less than 1% live births per cycle in women over the age of 40 years.

255. Polycystic ovarian syndrome (PCOS):
- **A.** is associated with a higher mean age at menarche.
- **B.** presents with primary amenorrhoea in under 1% of cases.
- **C.** commonly presents with virilization.
- **D.** is characterized by theca cell hypertrophy on histological examination of the ovaries.
- **E.** may be genetically determined.

256. Polycystic ovarian syndrome (PCOS) is associated with:

- **A.** decreased gonadotrophin-releasing hormone (GnRH) pulsatility.
- **B.** raised LH:FSH ratio.
- **C.** acanthosis nigricans.
- **D.** higher miscarriage rate.
- **E.** decreased hepatic production of sex hormone-binding globulin (SHBG).

257. Plasma gonadotrophin levels are raised in patients with:

- **A.** Kallmann's syndrome.
- **B.** anorexia nervosa.
- **C.** pituitary adenoma.
- **D.** Turner's syndrome.
- **E.** McCune-Albright syndrome.

258. The normal menstrual cycle is characterized by:

- **A.** basal LH levels higher than those of FSH during the early follicular phase.
- **B.** decreased frequency of GnRH pulses from the follicular to the luteal phase.
- **C.** an E_2 surge which precedes the LH surge by 12 hours.
- **D.** a fairly constant duration of the luteal phase.
- **E.** multiple follicular recruitment.

259. Kallmann's syndrome:

- **A.** has an equal incidence in males and females.
- **B.** is characterized by deficiency of all anterior pituitary hormones.
- **C.** is associated with colour blindness.
- **D.** can present as sexual infantilism.
- **E.** clinically mimics physiologically delayed puberty.

260. Craniopharyngioma:

- **A.** occurs almost exclusively in females.
- **B.** may present as primary amenorrhoea.
- **C.** may be associated with galactorrhoea.
- **D.** is commonly associated with calcification.
- **E.** commonly present clinically during the first decade of life.

261. Hyperprolactinaemia is associated with:

A. cimetidine.
B. methyl dopa.
C. metoclopramide.
D. chronic renal failure.
E. ovarian cysts.

262. Sheehan's syndrome:

A. usually results in isolated anterior pituitary dysfunction.
B. classically results from severe antepartum haemorrhage.
C. can occur up to 10 years after the index pregnancy.
D. is associated with a pituitary gland of normal size.
E. associated infertility is usually successfully treated with clomiphene citrate.

263. Prolactinomas:

A. in men are associated with oligospermia.
B. if untreated will progress from microadenoma to macro-adenoma.
C. are unlikely to recur following surgical excision.
D. could be treated with cabergoline.
E. are associated with an increased incidence of breast carcinoma.

264. Decreased hepatic synthesis of sex hormone-binding globulin (SHBG) is associated with:

A. testosterone.
B. insulin.
C. obesity.
D. the combined oral contraceptive pill.
E. gonadotrophin-releasing hormone (GnRH) analogues.

265. Late-onset congenital adrenal hyperplasia (CAH):

A. clinically presents with a picture similar to that of polycystic ovary syndrome.
B. is best diagnosed by measuring basal levels of 3α-androstanediol glucuronide.
C. due to 21-hydroxylase deficiency commonly presents with hypertension.
D. is inherited in an autosomal recessive mode.
E. is treated with low-dose dexamethasone.

266. With regard to androgen metabolism and effects in women:

- **A.** most (more than 90%) of circulating dehydroepiandrosterone sulphate (DHEAS) is of adrenal origin.
- **B.** less than 25% of women with polycystic ovaries (PCO) have increased levels of serum DHEAS.
- **C.** 17-hydroxyprogesterone is produced exclusively by the adrenals.
- **D.** rapid progression of hirsutism and/or virilization is suggestive of Cushing's syndrome.
- **E.** GnRH analogues may be used in the treatment of hyperandrogenism of adrenal origin.

267. With regard to premature ovarian failure (POF):

- **A.** the incidence is 5%.
- **B.** primary amenorrhoea is present in over 90% of cases.
- **C.** ovarian biopsy is essential to confirm the diagnosis.
- **D.** once the correct diagnosis has been made, spontaneous pregnancy cannot occur.
- **E.** it may be associated with hypothyroidism.

268. The following statements are correct with regard to the investigation of hirsutism:

- **A.** increased total testosterone concentration is probably due to adrenal hyperplasia.
- **B.** markedly raised dehydroepiandrosterone sulphate (DHAS) levels are suggestive of adrenal tumour.
- **C.** increased basal 17-hydroxyprogesterone levels are due to 17α-hydroxylase deficiency.
- **D.** increased 3α-androstanediol glucuronide is present in women with idiopathic hirsutism.
- **E.** deoxycortisol is increased in patients with 21-hydroxylase deficiency.

269. Medroxyprogesterone acetate (MPA), when used in the treatment of idiopathic hirsutism, works by:

- **A.** suppressing LH production.
- **B.** suppressing ovarian testosterone production.
- **C.** increasing the testosterone clearance rate.
- **D.** inhibiting 5α-reductase activity.
- **E.** increasing sex hormone-binding globulin (SHBG) production.

270. Precocious puberty:

A. may be secondary to a central nervous system tumour.
B. due to McCune-Albright syndrome is associated with low levels of gonadotrophins.
C. in the form of isolated premature thelarche is associated with advanced skeletal maturation.
D. in the form of premature adrenarche may be due to congenital adrenal hyperplasia.
E. treatment with cyproterone acetate (CPA) will lead to normal final height.

271. The following statements are correct with regard to precocious puberty:

A. the commonest cause in girls is idiopathic.
B. the commonest cause in boys is idiopathic.
C. may be due to primary hyperthyroidism.
D. GnRH analogues can improve the final height attained in girls with precocious puberty.
E. testolactone is effective treatment for gonadotrophin-independent precocious puberty.

272. Primary amenorrhoea due to:

A. congenital absence of the uterus is associated with normal breast development.
B. androgen insensitivity is associated with raised testosterone concentrations.
C. craniopharyngioma is associated with increased prolactin levels.
D. hypothalamopituitary failure may be associated with normal gonadotrophin levels.
E. hypothalamopituitary dysfunction is associated with withdrawal bleeding following a progesterone injection.

273. Primary amenorrhoea associated with poor breast development but normal uterus and lower genital tract may be due to:

A. Kallmann's syndrome.
B. testicular feminization syndrome.
C. polycystic ovary syndrome (PCOS).
D. Turner's syndrome.
E. 17α-hydroxylase deficiency.

274. Amenorrhoea:

A. due to hypothalamic dysfunction is associated with low plasma FSH and LH levels.
B. associated with markedly raised FSH concentration may be due to a pituitary tumour.
C. due to premature ovarian failure is always associated with increased FSH but normal LH levels.
D. due to pure gonadal dysgenesis is associated with 46,XY karyotype.
E. due to testicular feminization syndrome is associated with raised (male) levels of testosterone.

275. Clomiphene citrate is considered the first-line treatment of choice for ovulation induction in:

A. hypothalamopituitary dysfunction.
B. hypothalamopituitary failure.
C. anorexia nervosa.
D. primary hypothyroidism.
E. polycystic ovarian syndrome.

276. Gonadotrophin-releasing hormone (GnRH) analogues:

A. have a plasma half-life of 10 minutes.
B. lead to a hypo-oestrogenic state in most women after 4 days of treatment.
C. cause up to 10% loss of lumbar bone density after 6 months of treatment.
D. can help to correct preoperative anaemia before myomectomy.
E. improve fecundity in women with endometriosis.

277. A gonadotrophin-releasing hormone (GnRH) test is useful in the differential diagnosis of the following pubertal conditions:

A. McCune-Albright syndrome.
B. hypothalamic amenorrhoea.
C. hypopituitarism.
D. true precocious puberty.
E. granulosa cell ovarian tumour.

278. Amenorrhoea developing after stopping the combined oral contraceptive pill:

A. is more common following the use of pills with higher progestogen content.
B. is related to the length of its use.
C. may be due to hyperprolactinaemia.
D. may be due to polycystic ovarian syndrome.
E. should not be investigated before 12 months' duration, as spontaneous resumption of menses is the rule.

279. In polycystic ovary syndrome:

A. ovarian ultrasonography identifies 90% of women with clinical evidence of the disorder.
B. excess androgen is primarily derived from adrenal origin.
C. gonadotrophin-releasing hormone analogues may be used to treat hirsutism.
D. there is a recognized association with insulin resistance.
E. there is a recognized association with increased risk of ischaemic heart disease.

280. In seminal fluid analysis according to the WHO criteria:

A. teratozoospermia refers to more than 70% sperm with abnormal morphology.
B. 10,000 leucocytes per ml of semen is abnormal.
C. 5% of sperm coated with IgA sperm antibodies is abnormal.
D. a pH of 7.7 is abnormal.
E. normal results discriminate fertile from infertile men.

281. In the evaluation of the subfertile male:

A. a history of delayed sexual development and anosmia is suggestive of Klinefelter's syndrome.
B. a history of sinusitis and chronic bronchitis suggests Young's syndrome.
C. testicular size of 20 ml is indicative of testicular atrophy.
D. screening for the cystic fibrosis gene is indicated in patients with congenital absence of vas deferens.
E. testicular ultrasonography is of no value.

282. Oligozoospermia:

- **A.** is defined as a sperm concentration lower than 10 million per ml.
- **B.** is associated with the use of antiepileptic drugs.
- **C.** may be caused by sulphasalazine.
- **D.** is treatable with vitamin C.
- **E.** 2% of cases are associated with chromosomal abnormality.

283. Varicoceles:

- **A.** are found in 30–40% of men undergoing subfertility investigation.
- **B.** are bilateral in the majority of cases.
- **C.** may be associated with ipsilateral dull, aching sensation in the testicle, which is made worse by prolonged periods of standing.
- **D.** are found in approximately 5% of the general male population.
- **E.** raise testicular temperature.

284. Danazol:

- **A.** increases the hepatic synthesis of sex hormone-binding globulin (SHBG).
- **B.** is effective in the treatment of cyclic mastalgia.
- **C.** does not have any benefit above placebo in the treatment of premenstrual syndrome (PMS).
- **D.** can causes acne and oily skin.
- **E.** should be used in subfertile patients with minimal stage endometriosis.

285. Regarding genetic factors predisposing to recurrent abortion:

- **A.** 3% of couples in this category are balanced reciprocal translocation carriers.
- **B.** balanced translocations are more common if the previous pregnancy loss was associated with fetal malformation.
- **C.** new cytogenetic technology (such as banding techniques) have allowed detection of more subtle translocations.
- **D.** testicular biopsy is commonly performed to elucidate chromosome abnormalities in this group.
- **E.** detailed karyotyping of the abortus gives useful prognostic information for subsequent pregnancies.

286. Features of untreated Turner's syndrome (45,X) include:

A. low serum gonadotrophin levels.
B. low serum oestrogen levels.
C. hot flushes.
D. lymphoedema.
E. increased incidence of gonadal malignant tumours.

287. Drugs that can cause hirsutism include:

A. methyltestosterone.
B. phenytoin.
C. cyproterone acetate.
D. diazoxide.
E. danazol.

288. There is a recognized association between azoospermia and:

A. infection.
B. chemotherapy.
C. retrograde ejaculation.
D. testosterone administration.
E. varicocele.

289. Sperm suitable for intracytoplasmic sperm injection (ICSI) may be obtained in the following conditions:

A. Sertoli cell only syndrome.
B. congenital absence of the vas.
C. Klinefelter's syndrome.
D. following vasectomy.
E. following chemotherapy with alkylating agents to pre-pubertal males.

290. In anorexia nervosa:

A. the peak age of onset is usually between 20 and 25 years.
B. amenorrhoea is always preceded by severe weight loss.
C. there is severe wasting and marked distal weakness of limbs.
D. there is return of lanugo hair on the face and back.
E. there is usually a loss of secondary sexual characters.

291. In bulimia nervosa:
- **A.** regular menses occurs in only 5% of cases.
- **B.** patients are typically underweight.
- **C.** painless swelling of the parotid gland can occur.
- **D.** metabolic alkalosis may occur.
- **E.** acute gastric dilatation may occasionally occur.

292. Late-onset congenital adrenal hyperplasia:
- **A.** only presents in the homozygous state.
- **B.** is common amongst Ashkenazi Jews.
- **C.** may have raised follicular phase progesterone levels.
- **D.** is diagnosed by performing a short Synacthen test.
- **E.** is most appropriately treated by the combined oral contraceptive pill.

293. Testicular feminization (androgen insensitivity) syndrome is associated with:
- **A.** existence of ovarian and testicular tissue.
- **B.** ambiguous genitalia.
- **C.** 47,XX karyotype.
- **D.** hypoplastic breast.
- **E.** early onset of gonadal tumours.

294. The following drugs or conditions are paired with their effect on male fertility:
- **A.** reversible azoospermia : Salazopyrin.
- **B.** asthenozoospermia : Kartagener syndrome.
- **C.** retrograde ejaculation : diabetes mellitus.
- **D.** impotence : hyperprolactinaemia.
- **E.** absence of seminal fructose : congenital vasal agenesis.

Answers

240. ABC

The combination of secondary amenorrhoea, symptoms of oestrogen deficiency and raised gonadotrophins suggests the diagnosis of premature ovarian failure (POF). Up to 50% of women with POF have evidence of clinical autoimmune abnormalities (e.g. autoimmune thyroiditis, hypoparathyroidism, diabetes mellitus), of other collagen vascular disease (polyglandular autoimmune endocrine failure) or of circulating autoantibodies. Variations in X chromosome anomalies and its mosaics usually present as primary amenorrhoea, but some will achieve normal puberty and pregnancy too. Galactosaemia, an autosomal recessive deficiency of galactose-1-phosphate uridyltransferase, leads to local accumulation of galactose-1-phosphate and is associated with premature depletion of ovarian follicles.

Kallmann's syndrome is the most common cause of isolated gonadotrophin deficiency and is characterized by hypogonadotrophic hypogonadism (with or without anosmia). Laurence-Moon-Biedl syndrome is rare and presents as sexual infantilism (delayed puberty), associated with obesity, hypogonadism, learning disability, retinitis pigmentosa and abnormalities of digits. Both Kallmann's and Laurence-Moon-Biedl syndromes present with primary, rather than secondary, amenorrhoea.

241. BCD

Premature menopause is commonly defined as premature ovarian failure (POF) before the age of 40 years, and affects approximately 1% of women in that age group, totalling over 100,000 affected women in the UK. In most cases the condition is idiopathic with no identifiable cause. Recognized causes include chromosomal disorders (such as Turner's syndrome and pure gonadal dysgenesis), metabolic defects (17α-hydroxylase deficiency and galactosaemia), immunological disorders (Di George syndrome and ataxia telangiectasia), autoimmune diseases, infection (mumps oöphoritis and pelvic tuberculosis), and iatrogenic causes such as pelvic irradiation, ovarian surgery and chemotherapy. In general the diagnosis is based on a triad of amenorrhoea, raised gonadotrophin levels (particularly follicle-stimulating hormone) and symptoms of oestrogen deficiency. However, only about 50% of patients with POF will have hot flushes and genital atrophy. Some might not be amenorrhoeic, and may ovulate and menstruate sporadically.

242. ABE

SHBG is a glycoprotein that binds about 69% of circulating testosterone. Of the remaining testosterone, 30% is loosely bound to albumin and 1% is free (unbound); it is this unbound fraction that is responsible for the biological action of testosterone. Therefore, with the same level of serum testosterone, different levels of SHBG can lead to functional hyperandrogenaemia. Hyperthyroidism, pregnancy and oestrogen administration increase the level of SHBG, whereas corticoids, androgens, progestogens and growth hormone decrease the SHBG concentration. Circulating levels of SHBG are inversely related to weight and to insulin levels. The relationship between the levels of SHBG and insulin is so strong that SHBG concentration is a marker for hyperinsulinaemic insulin resistance, and a low level of SHBG is a predictor of future development of insulin-dependent diabetes mellitus.

243. BD

Prolactin is under the normal inhibitory control of dopamine, and hyperprolactinaemia can therefore be treated medically with dopamine agonists. Secondary causes of hyperprolactinaemia include hypothyroidism and drugs such as metoclopramide (dopamine antagonists) and phenothiazines. Some 20–25% of patients with acromegaly have pituitary tumours that secrete both growth hormone and prolactin. Having excluded 'secondary causes' of hyperprolactinaemia, all patients should have pituitary computed tomography and magnetic resonance imaging as up to 20% will have a non-functioning pituitary macroadenoma which causes hyperprolactinaemia because of stalk compression rather than secreting prolactin *per se*.

244. AC

Polycystic ovary syndrome (PCOS) is the commonest cause of anovulatory infertility. Ultrasonographic evidence of PCOS is found in about 20% of women in the reproductive age group. However, many of these women are asymptomatic and, if they are having regular periods, do not need treatment. A biochemical feature of PCOS is insulin resistance, i.e. reduced insulin sensitivity. Although many women are anovulatory and have low oestradiol levels, oestrone levels are normal or raised, which explains why such women have a withdrawal bleed following progesterone administration. Debate continues as to whether PCOS causes hyperprolactinaemia, but the large studies have consistently shown no change in mean levels from those in normal controls.

245. CDE

FSH stimulates follicular development in the ovary and spermatogenesis from Sertoli cells in the testis. Leydig cells secrete testosterone under the control of LH. FSH is under the inhibitory control of oestrogen and inhibin; levels are therefore high postmenopausally or in conditions associated with premature ovarian failure (e.g. Turner's syndrome). Levels are suppressed in patients with Cushing's syndrome, and this appears to be a direct effect of the glucocorticoids themselves. Long-term use of gonadotrophin-releasing hormone agonists suppresses LH and FSH levels.

246. BCD

DHAS reflects adrenal androgen secretion and is normal in over 50% of women with hirsutism. The underlying diagnosis is usually PCOS, and the best biochemical hallmark for the condition is a high circulating testosterone concentration (70% cases). Late-onset 21-hydroxylase deficiency may present as hirsutism and can indeed be excluded by a 17-hydroxyprogesterone basal follicular phase value of less than 5 nmol/l. Cyproterone acetate, not cyproheptadine, is an effective treatment.

247. ABCDE

Kallmann's syndrome is hypogonadotrophic hypogonadism associated with anosmia. Prader-Willi syndrome is another genetic defect characterized by hypotonia, short stature, obesity, learning disability and hypogonadism. Cirrhosis and haemochromatosis are recognized medical causes of hypogonadism; impaired liver oestrogen metabolism causes hypogonadism in cirrhotic males, and iron deposition in the gonads and liver causes hypogonadism in patients with haemochromatosis.

248. ADE

Precocious puberty can be classified as true (complete) or incomplete, and refers to the development of secondary sexual features before the age of 8 years in girls and 9 years in boys. Complete sexual precocity is usually constitutional and no underlying cause can be found. It refers simply to premature activation of the normal pubertal mechanism and can be successfully arrested with long-acting gonadotrophin-releasing hormone agonists. Hypothyroidism can be a cause, as can the McCune-Albright syndrome (triad of café au lait spots, fibrous dysplasia of bone, and precocious puberty). In contrast, incomplete sexual precocity is always caused by an autonomous secretion of hCG, LH or sex steroids. Causes include gonadotrophin-secreting tumours (teratomas, hepatomas), CNS germinomas, congenital adrenal hyperplasia and gonadal tumours.

249. BCE

Progesterone secreted from the corpus luteum is essential for the maintenance of the first 6 weeks of pregnancy, after which the fetoplacental unit takes over. Oestrogen does not appear to be essential for the maintenance of pregnancy at this stage. The fetal adrenal gland is large and secretes dehydroepiandrosterone (DHEA) which is aromatized in the placenta to oestrogen. Thus the principal source of maternal oestrogen is actually the fetal adrenal. Bilateral oöphorectomy during later pregnancy does not affect maternal oestrogen levels. There is epidemiological evidence that intrauterine growth restriction is associated with the subsequent development of hypertension, cardiovascular disease and diabetes in adult life.

250. E

Approximately 60% of circulating testosterone is bound to SHBG, the remainder to albumin. In contrast approximately 75% of progesterone is bound to albumin, 20% to corticosteroid-binding globulin and virtually none to SHBG. SHBG is increased in hyperthyroidism, cirrhosis and oestrogen therapy, but decreased in hypothyroidism, states of hyperandrogenism and by corticosteroids.

251. ABCDE

Glucocorticoid excess is a recognized cause of amenorrhoea. Galactosaemia is a cause of premature ovarian failure. Androgen insensitivity syndromes (e.g. testicular feminization) are due to defects in the androgen receptor; genetic males are phenotypically female, but present with primary amenorrhoea. 21-Hydroxylase deficiency results in amenorrhoea due to adrenal androgen excess. Craniopharyngiomas cause hypopituitarism.

252. AC

Clomiphene citrate is a weak oestrogen agonist which binds to hypothalamic oestrogen receptors, in competition with the potent oestradiol. As a result LH and FSH levels rise. Clomiphene is therefore ineffective in patients with pituitary disease or premature ovarian failure. The multiple pregnancy rate with clomiphene is about 8%. Recognized side-effects include visual disturbances, hot flushes, abdominal discomfort, nausea, vomiting, depression, insomnia, breast tenderness, weight gain, rashes, dizziness, hair loss and – as with other agents used for induction of ovulation – ovarian hyperstimulation syndrome.

253. ABCDE

The world's first IVF baby was born in 1978 in Oldham, England. Although IVF was first introduced as a treatment for tubal infertility, the indications have widened since then, and now it has a place in the treatment of almost all causes of infertility. Tubal disease, however, remains the single most common female indication, followed by unexplained infertility. According to the UK Human Fertilization and Embryology Authority (HFEA), tubal disease was recorded in 43% and unexplained infertility in 37.8% of the 24,708 IVF cycles performed in the UK during 1994. In premature ovarian failure the only proven treatment is IVF using donor eggs.

254. CD

According to the UK HFEA, the live birth rate per IVF cycle (often referred to as the take-home-baby rate) using the woman's own eggs was 14.2% in 1994. There were three principal factors affecting this rate: sperm defect, the woman's age and her past obstetric history. In the presence of male factor infertility there was a lower rate of fertilization, and hence fewer embryos available for transfer. The live birth rate decreased with advancing woman's age: 17.3% under the age of 25 years, 17.2% between 25 and 29 years, 16% between 30 and 34 years, 12.3% between 35 and 39 years, 5.4% between 40 and 44 years, and 2.4% at age 45 years and over. Women who have had a previous pregnancy (regardless of its outcome) had a live birth rate of 18% (as opposed to 14.2% for all women). Those with a previous live birth had a LBR of 24%; if that live birth resulted from a previous IVF attempt, the live birth rate increased to 30%. Although it was originally thought that women with tubal infertility would have a higher success rate with IVF than those with other causes, this was found not to be correct in any of the world's large series, and it is now accepted that the female indication is not a principal factor affecting the live birth rate.

255. DE

PCOS is a complex heterogeneous disorder with diverse clinical and biochemical features. The following organs and systems are proposed to contribute to the pathogenesis of PCOS: the hypothalamopituitary unit, the ovary, the adrenal gland, the skin and insulin resistance. Women with PCOS have a similar mean age at menarche (12–13 years) to that of normal women. The condition should be considered in the differential diagnosis of primary amenorrhoea because 10% of patients present with this complaint. Virilization is the least common symptom of PCOS (infertility, hirsutism and amenorrhoea being the commonest) and a more serious cause, such as androgen-producing ovarian or adrenal tumours, should be looked for. Familial clustering of PCOS suggests the possibility of genetic transmission, but the available evidence does not support simple mendelian transmission. There seems to be a complex mode of transmission, preferentially through the maternal line, with the male variant presenting as premature (at less than age 30 years) bitemporal balding.

256. BCDE

PCOS is associated with increased GnRH pulsatility, which contributes to the preferential increase in plasma LH levels. Although an increased LH:FSH ratio is a common feature, 20% of women with PCOS have a normal LH:FSH ratio. Acanthosis nigricans is a condition involving localized skin areas of velvety grey-brown hyperpigmentation seen in women with PCOS and insulin resistance resulting from chronic hyperinsulinaemia. A higher miscarriage rate has been documented in women with PCOS, particularly those with chronically raised plasma LH levels. Androgen excess leads to inhibition of SHBG production, resulting in increased free androgen levels.

257. D

Gonadotrophin levels are suppressed in females with Kallmann's syndrome, anorexia nervosa and McCune-Albright syndrome. They are normal or suppressed in women who have pituitary adenoma and raised in those with Turner's syndrome (ovarian failure).

258. BDE

The normal menstrual cycle is characterized by early rise of both gonadotrophins, but FSH levels are higher than those of LH. GnRH pulses are more frequent (every 60–90 minutes) and of lower amplitude during the follicular phase, compared with the less frequent (120–180 minutes) and higher-amplitude pulses during the luteal phase. The E_2 surge usually precedes the LH surge by 12 hours and the latter is suggested to stimulate the second meiotic division. Variation in the length of the menstrual cycle is due to variation in the follicular phase, the luteal phase being fairly constant at about 14 days. Multiple follicular recruitment and development is the rule, but only one follicle reaches the stage of ovulation while the other follicles undergo atresia.

259. CDE

Hypogonadal eunuchoidism or Kallmann's syndrome is the most common cause of isolated gonadotrophin deficiency.

The familial occurrence of Kallmann's syndrome is characterized by hypogonadotrophic hypogonadism, in association with anosmia, colour blindness and learning disability. Although it is diagnosed in both sexes, the male:female ratio is 11:1. In absence of other congenital anomalies, the syndrome is usually identified at the age of puberty (which is absent) and presents as sexual infantilism. Blood levels of FSH, LH, E_2 (female) and testosterone (male) are very low. In the absence of olfactory defect (anosmia) or other anomalies mentioned above, the main differential diagnosis of Kallmann's syndrome is from physiologically delayed puberty.

260. BCD

Craniopharyngioma are cysts derived from the remnants of Rathke's pouch. These tumours occur in both sexes but are commoner in men, with the highest prevalence during the second decade. They commonly present clinically around the age of puberty. The commonest clinical presentation is visual field defects in addition to varying degrees of panhypopituitarism. The degree of hypothalamopituitary impairment depends on the extent of pituitary stalk involvement and thus craniopharyngioma may present as primary amenorrhoea or other trophic hormone deficiency with or without galactorrhoea. These tumours are commonly associated with calcification and are readily recognizable on lateral skull radiographs.

261. ABCD

The commonest cause of functional hyperprolactinaemia is drug induced. Medications that interfere with dopamine synthesis, release or reuptake are associated with increased prolactin secretion. Chronic renal failure is associated with hyperprolactinaemia which is normalized following transplantation, but not haemodialysis. Ovarian cysts do not cause hyperprolactinaemia, although approximately 20% of women with polycystic ovary syndrome have increased prolactin levels.

262. C

Sheehan's syndrome is hypopituitarism due to infarction resulting from hypovolaemic shock secondary to massive postpartum haemorrhage, presumably because of the increased vascularity and growth of the pituitary that occur during pregnancy in response to oestrogen. The degree of hypopituitarism is highly variable. Posterior pituitary function is usually affected; however, overt symptoms of diabetes insipidus are uncommon. The following pituitary functions are affected in order of frequency: growth hormone, gonadotrophins, thyroid-stimulating hormone and adrenocorticotrophic hormone. Although acute hypopituitarism may occur, it is more common for the syndrome to develop slowly and the diagnosis may be made 10–15 years after the obstetric incident. The pituitary gland is smaller in women with Sheehan's syndrome, as shown by significantly smaller sellar volume on magnetic resonance imaging. Fertility can be achieved in these women by means of human menopausal gonadotrophins, human chorionic gonadotrophin and other hormone replacement as necessary. The successful use of clomiphene citrate requires intact pituitary function, which is not the case in Sheehan's syndrome.

263. DE

Hyperprolactinaemic men will seek medical advice because of impaired libido, sexual impotence and/or visual and neurological symptoms, if hyperprolactinaemia is due to pituitary tumour. Microadenomas do not necessarily progress to macroadenomas and their natural history is still unknown. In fact some microadenomas are reported to disappear with long-term follow-up. Approximately 50% (range 20–80%) of patients will later develop hyperprolactinaemia following surgery. Although a substantial proportion of patients with hyperprolactinaemia will have a prolactinoma, the possibility of non-functioning tumours compressing the pituitary stalk (particularly in the presence of only moderately raised prolactin levels) should be considered.

264. ABC

Androgens decrease hepatic synthesis of SHBG, which in turn increases their biological availability by raising the level of free testosterone (i.e. inducing a positive feedback loop). Obesity, which is commoner in women with polycystic ovaries (PCO), is known to decrease SHBG activity independent of the presence of PCO. Insulin also decreases the hepatic synthesis SHBG, independent of testosterone, i.e. SHBG concentration is inversely proportional to insulin resistance when corrected for obesity and testosterone effects. Oestrogens increase

SHBG and thus the oral contraceptive pill is used to treat hirsutism. GnRH analogues do not directly affect SHBG concentration; however, if used to treat hirsutism, ovarian androgen production is inhibited, and thus they may contribute (indirectly) to increased hepatic synthesis of SHBG.

265. ADE

CAH is due to an enzyme defect in the adrenal cortex leading to excessive androgen production. The commonest enzyme defect is 21-hydroxylase (p450c21). A significantly raised early morning (basal) level of 17-hydroxyprogesterone is diagnostic of late-onset CAH. If basal levels are normal or borderline in women with suspected CAH, adrenocorticotrophic hormone (ACTH) stimulation may be used and 17-hydroxyprogesterone concentration is measured again. Hypertension is a feature of CAH due to 11-hydroxylase deficiency.

Whereas testosterone is the major circulating androgen, dihydrotestosterone (DHT) is the major nuclear androgen in target tissues. The enzyme 5α-reductase converts testosterone and androstenedione into DHT. 3α-Androstanediol is the peripheral tissue metabolite of DHT, and its glucuronide, 3α-androstanediol glucuronide (3α-AG) is the most sensitive marker of peripheral (cellular) metabolism of androgens and correlates with 5α-reductase activity. 3α-AG concentration is raised in women with hirsutism even if testosterone levels are normal. However, its measurement does not affect the clinical management of cases of hirsutism and, hence, it is not measured in routine clinical practice. In addition, the normal and abnormal values overlap by about 20%.

266. A

DHEAS is considered the best marker of adrenal androgen production and approximately 50% of women with PCO have raised serum levels of DHEAS, suggestive of adrenal gland contribution to their hyperandrogenism. 17-Hydroxyprogesterone is produced by both the ovary and adrenal but its raised early morning value is suggestive of the diagnosis of adult-onset congenital adrenal hyperplasia. Rapid progression of hirsutism and/or virilization should always arouse the suspicion of an ovarian or adrenal neoplasia. GnRH analogues are fairly effective in the treatment of hyperandrogenism of ovarian origin (being gonadotrophin dependent), but not that of adrenal origin (ACTH dependent).

267. E

POF is reported in 1% of women less than 40 years old; it is associated with primary and secondary amenorrhoea in 25% and 75% of affected women, respectively. Ovarian biopsy is unnecessary and can be misleading in women with POF, because absence of ovarian follicles in the biopsy does not correlated with the clinical outcome. POF, particularly if associated with secondary amenorrhoea, is not uncommonly followed by episodes of normal menses, ovulation and even spontaneous pregnancy. Up to 50% of cases of POF are associated with autoimmunity and circulating autoantibodies, and POF is reported to occur in women with autoimmune disease, most commonly hypothyroidism due to autoimmune thyroiditis.

268. BDE

Increased total testosterone concentration is often due to ovarian hyperandrogenism (e.g. PCOS). Although adrenal hyperplasia due to 21-hydroxylase deficiency may also cause an increased total testosterone concentration, these women will also have raised 17-hydroxyprogesterone levels.

Most DHAS is of adrenal origin and, if levels are two times or more than the upper limit of the normal range, adrenal tumour should be excluded. 21-Hydroxylase deficiency (and not 17-hydroxylase) is associated with raised levels of basal 17-hydroxyprogesterone.

In women with hirsutism and regular ovulatory cycles, determination of raised circulating 3α-androstanediol glucuronide levels confirms the diagnosis of idiopathic hirsutism (due to increased androgen metabolism at the target tissue). However, as this finding does not affect clinical management and there is some overlap between normal and abnormal values, this assay is not used in routine clinical practice.

269. ABC

In women with idiopathic hirsutism in whom the combined pill (the first choice of treatment) is contraindicated or unwanted, MPA is used with similar results. It inhibits LH production and hence ovarian testosterone production. It also increases the rate of testosterone clearance from the circulation. Although it inhibits SHBG production, which has the potential knock-on effect of increasing free testosterone levels, the decreased production of testosterone is much greater, with the overall effect of reducing free testosterone levels. It is given in a dose of 150 mg intramuscularly every 3 months, or 30 mg/day orally.

270. ABD

McCune-Albright syndrome is a form of gonadotrophin-independent precocious puberty. It is associated with cystic ovaries that produce oestradiol and thus involves low (or normal) gonadotrophin levels. Skeletal maturation is appropriate for age in girls with premature thelarche but advanced in those with central precocious puberty. In premature adrenarche, follow-up is essential because progressive or extensive virilization warrants further investigations to rule out congenital adrenal hyperplasia or adrenal tumour. CPA arrests the development of secondary sex characteristics effectively, but does not increase the final height attained.

271. ADE

The first detectable endocrine manifestation of puberty in both sexes is a nocturnal increase in the amplitude of LH secretion in response to an increase in the pulsatile secretion of GnRH. Idiopathic precocious puberty is the commonest cause (90%) in girls; however, in boys it is almost always secondary to a lesion in the central nervous system, such as a tumour. Primary hypothyroidism (not hyperthyroidism) may cause precocious puberty, which is characterized by isolated breast development and without the recognized pubertal growth pattern. In contrast to other conventional therapy (e.g. cyproterone acetate and long-acting progesterone), GnRH analogues improve the final height, although they do not restore it to the parental centile. Testolactone, a peripheral aromatase inhibitor, is used to decrease steroid production in girls with gonadotrophin-independent precocious puberty.

272. ABCDE

Two conditions are associated with an absent or rudimentary uterus: congenital absence of the uterus and androgen insensitivity syndrome; the latter is associated with 'male' levels of plasma testosterone. Craniopharyngioma, like other pituitary tumours, may interfere with dopamine release (as a result of pituitary stalk compression) and thus may present with primary amenorrhoea ± other trophic hormone deficiency ± galactorrhoea. In hypothalamopituitary failure, and particularly pituitary failure, gonadotrophin levels are either low or in the low normal range. The diagnosis is established by the finding of hypogonadism, other trophic hormone deficiency and imaging techniques. Positive withdrawal bleeding confirms the presence of an oestrogenized endometrium in several conditions (e.g. PCOS and hypothalamopituitary dysfunction).

273. ADE

Absent breast development signifies absence of (past or present) exposure to oestrogens. Hypogonadotrophic hypogonadism is one of the most common causes of primary amenorrhoea. In Kallmann's syndrome, in addition to anosmia, patients also have an anomaly of the normal regulation of quantitative or qualitative gonadotrophin-releasing hormone (GnRH) secretion. GnRH testing should be used to differentiate hypothalamic origin from pituitary origin of hypogonadotrophic hypogonadism. Testicular feminization (androgen insensitivity) syndrome is associated with well-developed breasts and absent uterus. In PCOS, although a recognized cause of primary amenorrhoea, patients are well oestrogenized and the condition is associated with normal breast development. Turner's syndrome (and its mosaic variants) is associated with hypergonadotrophic hypogonadism (raised FSH levels). Therefore, patients with primary amenorrhoea and increased FSH concentration should be karyotyped. 17α-Hydroxylase enzyme (present in both ovary and adrenals) is essential for the sex steroid and corticosteroid pathways. Patients with 17α-hydroxylase deficiency and 46,XX karyotype present with hypertension, hypokalaemia, high plasma progesterone levels and raised FSH and LH concentrations.

274. BDE

Hypothalamic dysfunction (due to weight loss, exercise, etc.) is associated with normal plasma levels of FSH and LH. However, it may be associated with abnormal LH (and thus GnRH) pulsatility. Although the commonest cause of raised

FSH concentration is gonadal failure, the finding of markedly increased FSH levels in the presence of normal circulating oestradiol (with or without pressure symptoms) should alert the clinician to the rare possibility of gonadotrophin-secreting adenoma. Typically, premature ovarian failure is associated with markedly raised FSH and LH levels (similar to natural menopause); however, it is not uncommon to find variable endocrine features such as high FSH and normal LH levels, or even normal FSH, LH and oestradiol concentrations too.

Patients with pure gonadal dysgenesis have 46,XX or 46,XY karyotype, bilateral streak gonads and usually do not have the physical stigma of Turner's syndrome. Following puberty, they present with sexual infantilism, eunuchoid features and raised serum levels of FSH and LH. Females with testicular feminization syndrome are genetic males (46,XY), have testes and thus their plasma testosterone level is in the normal male range.

275. AE

Clomiphene citrate is expected to be successful in inducing ovulation only when there is an 'adequate' concentration of circulating oestradiol (E_2) as demonstrated by: eumenorrhoea or oligomenorrhoea, plasma E_2 level greater than 50 pg/ml, or positive withdrawal bleeding in response to progestogen challenge testing. Therefore, clomiphene citrate is the first-line ovulation-inducing agent in hypothalamopituitary dysfunction and polycystic ovarian syndrome. In hypothalamo-pituitary failure and anorexia nervosa there is E_2 lack and thus clomiphene will not be successful in inducing ovulation. Primary hypothyroidism may cause anovulation due to associated hyperprolactinaemia. Hormone replacement (thyroxine) should be the treatment of first choice.

276. CD

GnRH analogues are synthesized by substituting amino acids at positions 6 and 10 of the original decapeptide GnRH. Therefore, they have a longer plasma half-life (greater than 2 hours) because of their resistance to endopeptidases and decreased metabolic clearance. During the first few days of treatment there is a flare-up effect, with raised gonadotrophin (and oestrogen) levels. However, most women will be hypo-oestrogenic within 2–3 weeks of starting treatment. The profound hypo-oestrogenism induced by GnRH analogues will affect virtually all patients treated, resulting in a significant reduction in trabecular bone density after 24 weeks of treatment, which may not be reversible in some women.

By inducing amenorrhoea and hypomenorrhoea, GnRH analogues are useful in women scheduled to have myomectomy, as menstrual blood loss is decreased so improving anaemia. Although a GnRH analogue-induced hypo-oestrogenic state can improve the symptoms in women with endometriosis, there is no scientific evidence that fecundity is improved in these patients.

277. BCD

GnRH (100 mg subcutaneously or intramuscularly) is used for the GnRH test. Plasma FSH, LH ($\pm$ oestradiol) are measured before the injection (time 00.00 hours) and at 0.30, 1.00 and 1.30 hours. The GnRH test helps to differentiate hypothalamic from pituitary origin in cases of delayed puberty or primary amenorrhoea of hypothalamopituitary origin. It is also useful to confirm the diagnosis in cases of true (central) precocious puberty.

McCune-Albright syndrome will usually be diagnosed by its characteristic features of polyosteotic fibrous dysplasia, cutaneous pigmentation, precocious puberty and ovarian cysts on pelvic ultrasonography. Granulosa cell ovarian tumour is a rare cause of gonadotrophin-independent precocious puberty, and presents with a pelvic mass diagnosed on pelvic ultrasonography.

278. CD

The term 'post-pill amenorrhoea' (PPA) describes amenorrhoea that develops after stopping the combined oral contraceptive pill. The term is purely descriptive and should not imply any causal association; such an association has never been proven. Large-scale population-based studies have shown that amenorrhoea longer than 3 months occurs in 3.3%, and that for longer than 6 months in 1.8%, of the population; an incidence similar to that of PPA. Most women in the reproductive age group should have normal menstrual cycles within 6 months of discontinuation of the pill. Any amenorrhoea persisting for more than 6 months should be investigated. As expected, pregnancy should first be excluded.

Oral contraceptive pill users are not 'immune' to the development of pituitary adenoma or PCOS, and these too, amongst other causes, have to be excluded.

279. CDE

Ovarian ultrasonography identifies only 50% of women with clinical and biochemical evidence of PCOS, and thus may not be used as the only diagnostic criterion. Although adrenal androgen contribution in PCOS is well documented, in vivo studies have uniformly shown increased secretion of ovarian androgens with suppression by GnRH analogues or oral contraceptive pill administration. Therefore, GnRH analogues have been used effectively to treat hirsutism due to increased ovarian androgen levels, as in PCOS.

Polycystic ovaries are associated with several conditions known to cause insulin resistance and diabetes mellitus: Cushing's syndrome, types A and B insulin resistance, and obesity. Furthermore, obese women with PCOS are more likely to have hyperinsulinaemia, which correlates negatively with high density lipoprotein 2 (HDL-2) concentrations. This suggests that hyperinsulinaemic women with PCOS may have an increased risk of ischaemic heart disease as circulating HDL-2 is thought to be protective against the development of atheroma.

280. A

WHO criteria for a normal semen include: volume = 2 ml or more, pH 7.2–7.8, sperm concentration 20 million per ml or more, motility 50% or greater with forward progression, morphology 30% or more normal forms, 10% or less of sperm coated with sperm antibodies (using immuno-bead test). It is important to remember that WHO criteria do not discriminate 'fertile' from 'infertile' men. Spontaneous pregnancy can occur as long as sperm are present, although the lower the count the lower the fecundity.

281. BD

A history of delayed sexual development and anosmia suggests Kallmann's syndrome. Klinefelter's syndrome is 47,XXY. Young's syndrome (epididymal obstruction associated with chronic sinopulmonary infections) usually presents with azoospermia. Although there is some variation with race, normal testis size is greater than 19 ml. Testicular ultrasonography can diagnose ejaculatory duct obstruction, small varicoceles, locate impalpable testes and facilitate detection of cysts or other abnormalities in the scrotum. Some 40% or more of men with congenital absence of vas deferens are carriers of cystic fibrosis gene mutations and, therefore, require specific screening and counselling.

282. BCE

Oligozoospermia (according to the WHO criteria) is sperm concentration less than 20 million per ml. Hyposexuality and poor semen quality are common in epileptic men. The aetiology is multifactorial and includes a direct effect of antiepileptic drugs on the testes. For example, carbamazepine is secreted in semen in high concentration and inhibits testosterone synthesis by the Leydig cells in vitro. There is no proof that vitamin C is of any value in the treatment of male subfertility.

283. ACE

The incidence of varicocele in the general population has been estimated at about 15% but appears to be higher (up to 40%) in subfertile couples. Varicocele has been associated with abnormalities in semen parameters and implicated as a cause of male subfertility for many years. Impaired blood drainage from the testis leading to increased scrotal temperature with its deleterious effect on spermatogenesis has been proposed as its main aetiology. The majority of varicoceles are unilateral and located on the left side.

284. BD

Danazol is used in the treatment of conditions that respond to the reduction in gonadal steroid activity. It suppresses the mid-cycle LH and FSH surges, reduces LH pulsatility, and inhibits ovarian responsiveness and steroidogenesis. At a dose of 100–400 mg/day over 2–4 months, danazol relieves the pain and tenderness of severe cyclical mastalgia. Improvement is likely to be sustained for several months after treatment. It has also been used in the treatment of PMS, and controlled trials have shown a superior effect to placebo. The androgenic side-effects of danazol are at least partly due to its effect on the level of SHBG, which is reduced by direct inhibition of its hepatic synthesis. These side-effects include acne, oily skin and increased facial hair. Brunette patients have a higher incidence of these problems than those with blond hair. There is no evidence that the use of danazol in subfertile patients with minimal endometriosis is of any benefit in increasing the pregnancy rate. In fact, patients taking danazol should use reliable contraception (to avoid virilization of the female fetus), and as such the drug has a detrimental effect by delaying pregnancy.

285. ABCE

A few chromosome abnormalities resulting in spontaneous abortion arise from structural chromosome abnormalities in the parents. The most common of these are balanced translocations. Translocation describes a situation in which a fragment of one chromosome becomes attached to the broken end of another. These may be reciprocal involving two chromosomes in mutual exchange of broken off fragments or Robertsonian, in which the translocation involves two acrocentric chromosomes. Karyotypic examinations in couples who have had recurrent spontaneous miscarriages reveal an approximate 3% incidence of balanced reciprocal translocations. This incidence increased to 13.6% in couples with a history of miscarriage plus a fetal abnormality. The introduction of chromosome banding techniques and new technologies such as in situ hybridization are more likely to identify small translocation areas. This may be true in part for the increasing incidence of these karyotypic abnormalities in more contemporary series. Some studies have shown that testicular biopsies in male partners of women who had multiple spontaneous abortions had, in some circumstances, abnormalities of meiosis even though the blood karyotype was normal. However, this is an invasive test that is not often utilized.

When karyotyping of two successive abortuses is performed, a correlation is found between normal and abnormal characters in the two specimens. Studies have indicated that, if the first abortus is chromosomally normal, the second abortus has at least a 66% chance of being chromosomally normal. If the first abortus is chromosomally abnormal, there is a 75% chance that the second will be abnormal. There is thus prognostic information to be gained in performing karyotyping on the abortus material. If a patient is a balanced translocation carrier, there is obviously no treatment for the condition. However, amniocentesis or chorionic villus sampling may be offered.

286. BD

In Turner's syndrome there is hypergonadotrophic hypogonadism. Despite low oestrogen levels, these women do not have hot flushes: only after oestrogen is administered and withdrawn do they experience hot flushes. The incidence of gonadal malignant tumours is increased only where there is a Y chromosome in the karyotype (e.g. mosaic 45,X/46,XY).

287. ABDE

Cyproterone acetate is an antiandrogen used in the treatment of hirsutism. It also has progestational activity and is a component of some combined oral contraceptive pills (e.g. Dianette).

288. ABCD

Causes of azoospermia (no spermatozoa in the ejaculate) can be classified into obstructive and non-obstructive. The latter are usually due to testicular failure, but can rarely be due to hypogonadotrophic hypogonadism. Infection can cause occlusion of the vas deferens. Chemotherapy, especially with alkylating agents and when combined with radiotherapy, causes destruction of the germ calls, thereby causing testicular failure. Retrograde ejaculation, when complete, classically presents with aspermia (no ejaculate). When partial, it usually presents with oligozoospermia, but may present with azoospermia. The clue to this diagnosis is a very low ejaculate volume (less than 0.5 ml). Testosterone therapy, although a possible treatment for impotence due to low testosterone levels, actually inhibits spermatogenesis through its negative feedback effect on LH and FSH levels. Varicocele may be associated with teratoasthenozoospermia. Having said that, it is important to recognize that there is no prospective controlled evidence that surgical treatment of varicocele leads to a significant improvement in pregnancy rate.

289. ABCDE

In conventional in vitro fertilization (IVF), where the sperm is incubated with the oöcytes, about 50,000 to 100,000 sperm are needed per oöcyte to achieve fertilization. ICSI involves the microinjection of a single sperm into the oöcyte to achieve fertilization. It is used to overcome severe male factor infertility where there are very few sperm available, or even when there is azoospermia, when the sperm used for ICSI could be obtained through testicular biopsy or fine-needle aspiration. The sperm characteristics do not seem to be important to success following ICSI.

In all conditions listed in the question, pregnancies have been reported following treatment with ICSI. Sperm can be retrieved relatively easily in obstructive cases such as absence of the vas and following vasectomy. However, it is important to recognize that there is an association between congenital bilateral absence of the vas (CBAV) and cystic fibrosis carrier status; before embarking on ICSI for CBAV, the patient should be screened for cystic fibrosis and counselled accordingly.

In cases of Sertoli cell only syndrome it was originally thought that the disorder was present throughout the whole testicular tissue. However, the concept of 'focality' is now well recognized, where there are foci of normal spermatogenesis in the testis from which sperm for ICSI could be obtained. In some cases of testicular failure, even when the FSH concentration is over 25 IU/l, sperm have been retrieved and pregnancies using ICSI reported.

290. D

Anorexia nervosa is at least ten times more common in women than men. Its peak age of onset is between 14 and 17 years of age, when the girl is usually first aware of her body image, but it occasionally affects prepupertal or mature adult females. Amenorrhoea may be the first symptom, or may occur at a later stage following severe weight loss. There is severe wasting and severe proximal weakness of limbs. Lanugo, a fine downy hair, normal in childhood, returns and is most prominent on the face, forearms, nape of the neck and down the spine. Secondary sexual characters, including hair, are preserved.

291. CDE

Some 40–95% of bulimic women have menstrual irregularities. However, female psychiatric inpatients have amenorrhoea at rate of 27%. Bulimic patients are usually of average weight but can be underweight or overweight by variable degrees. Recurrent vomiting causes painless swelling of the parotid glands, hoarseness of voice and dental caries. Gastrointestinal reflux may be a problem and occasionally acute dilatation of the stomach may occur. Electrolyte disturbances with low serum potassium and raised bicarbonate levels may be present, giving a hypokalaemic alkalosis.

292. BCD

The main symptoms are related to hyperandrogenism. These occur more commonly in the homozygous state, but can also occur in the heterozygous form. It is one of the commonest autosomal recessive conditions, with a high prevalence amongst Ashkenazi Jews (1 in 30), Hispanics (1 in 40), and Yugoslavs (1 in 50). The condition is diagnosed by stimulating the pituitary adrenal axis by giving synthetic ACTH (Synacthen). If there is a block at the 21-hydroxylase enzyme, then 21-hydroxyprogesterone (21-OHP) is not converted to 17-hydroxypregnenolone, and 21-OHP levels are raised. Other enzyme defects are 3β-hydroxysteroid dehydrogenase and, rarely, 11β-hydroxylase deficiency. Progesterone levels are raised as it is a substrate for the 21-hydroxylase enzyme. Treatment is specific and is with glucocorticoids.

293. All answers are false

Testicular feminization (complete androgen insensitivity) is a condition in which there is congenital insensitivity to androgens due to a deficiency in the androgen intracellular receptors. The chromosomal complement is 46,XY. Affected individuals have subsequent development of the external genitalia along female lines. Androgen induction of Wolffian duct development also does not occur. Development of müllerian duct is suppressed as gonads retain Müllerian inhibiting factor (MIF) activity. Sex assignment is uniformly female. There are no traces of androgen activity or sexual ambiguity. Testes may be present in the abdominal cavity, inguinal canal or labia. Normal breast development occurs. In contrast to other intersex condition with a Y chromosome, gonadal tumours tend to occur relatively late. Therefore, gonadectomy can usually be deferred until after puberty to permit oestrogen production and the development of secondary sexual characteristics. The syndrome is transmitted through an X-linked recessive trait. Apparent sisters of affected persons will have a one in three chance of being XY. A female offspring of a normal female who is a sister of an affected person has a one in six chance of being XY.

294. ABCDE

Drug history is of particular importance in clinical assessment of male infertility. Salazopyrin, used for treatment of ulcerative colitis, is known to cause reversible azoospermia. Other drugs with adverse effects on spermatogenesis are cytotoxic or immunosuppressive agents, antihypertensives, nitrofurantoin, anabolic steroids, nicotine, alcohol and other drugs of habituation. Hyperprolactinaemia may be associated with diminished libido and potency, whereas diabetes mellitus may cause retrograde ejaculation through the associated neuropathy. In Kartagener's syndrome there may be absent cilia, which may be also responsible for bronchiectasis and asthenozoospermia.

5

Medical and Surgical Gynaecology

Questions

295. The use of prophylactic low-dose heparin in a patient undergoing major gynaecological surgery is associated with:

A. a reduced risk of thromboembolism.
B. an increase in the incidence of abdominal wound haematoma.
C. an increase in blood transfusion requirements.
D. a significant drop in postoperative haemoglobin concentration.
E. the development of osteoporosis.

296. Features of Turner's syndrome (45,X) include:

A. absent vagina.
B. coarctation of the aorta.
C. kyphoscoliosis.
D. increasing incidence with advanced maternal age.
E. cubitus valgus.

297. In a medicolegal claim, negligence is always proven if there is:

A. a retained swab.
B. an elective operative procedure without informed consent.
C. failed sterilization.
D. an admission of error by the clinician.
E. a dural tap after epidural anaesthesia.

298. Dilatation and curettage (D&C) is indicated in the investigation of:

A. infertility.
B. menorrhagia in a 37-year-old woman.
C. persistent intermenstrual bleeding in a 29-year-old woman.
D. postmenopausal bleeding.
E. suspected pelvic tuberculosis.

299. In the treatment of uncomplicated vaginal candidiasis:

A. cure rates are about 80–90%.
B. short (1-day) courses are just as effective as longer ones.
C. oral treatment may be preferable where there is pronounced vulval inflammation.
D. pessaries may cause condom or diaphragm failure.
E. oral fluconazole treatments are safe in pregnancy.

300. Recurrent vaginal candidiasis is associated with:

A. reinfection from the anus or rectum.
B. sexual transmission from the male partner.
C. the combined oral contraceptive pill containing 30 μg ethinyloestradiol.
D. broad-spectrum antibiotics.
E. iron and/or zinc deficiency.

301. In bacterial vaginosis:

A. the causative organism has been identified as *Gardnerella vaginalis.*
B. the predominant symptom is vaginal discharge.
C. the vaginal pH is usually greater than 5.0–5.5.
D. 30–40% of women are asymptomatic.
E. the mode of transmission is often sexual intercourse.

302. Atrophic vaginitis:

A. occurs only after the menopause.
B. is usually symptomatic.
C. can be confirmed by vaginal cytology.
D. is treated by local steroids.
E. is a recognized cause of postmenopausal bleeding.

303. Common changes in diethlyl stilboestrol (DES) exposed females offspring include:
- **A.** clear-cell adenocarcinoma of the lower genital tract.
- **B.** transverse vaginal and cervical ridges.
- **C.** pseudopolyps and 'Cockscomb' cervix.
- **D.** vaginal adenosis.
- **E.** cervical stenosis.

304. In surgery for prolapse:
- **A.** sacral colpopexy for enterocele attaches the vault of vagina to the sacral periosteum.
- **B.** Manchester repair differs from the Fothergill procedure as it includes anterior repair.
- **C.** in Manchester repair, the cervix is transected at the level of the internal os.
- **D.** amputation of the cervix is not part of the Le Fort procedure.
- **E.** transvaginal sacrospinous colpopexy can involve a midline vertical cut in the posterior vaginal wall.

305. In vaginal hysterectomy for prolapse:
- **A.** the uterosacral and cardinal ligaments are usually taken as one pedicle.
- **B.** the peritoneal cavity must be opened before taking the cardinal ligament.
- **C.** oöphorectomy is easier than in an abdominal procedure.
- **D.** the ovarian ligament should be spared if the ovaries are conserved.
- **E.** subsequent enterocele is more common than after the Manchester repair.

306. The following statements are correct with regard to lasers:
- **A.** LASER stands for Light Absorption by Stimulated Emission of Radiation.
- **B.** laser cone biopsy specimens give better histology at the specimen margin than diathermy loop.
- **C.** laser excision of vulval intraepithelial neoplasia (VIN) is less painful than local excision.
- **D.** laser is probably the treatment of choice for isolated vaginal intraepithelial neoplasia (VAIN).
- **E.** the neodymium yttrium-aluminium-garnet (NdYAG) laser is superior to the carbon dioxide laser for incision of tissues.

307. In total abdominal hysterectomy (TAH):

A. the ovarian ligament is cut if the ovary is to be removed.
B. if the ureter is damaged, the damage occurs most commonly at the uterine artery pedicle.
C. the ureter is found running at right angles to the broad ligament at its base.
D. the dome of the bladder is fixed to the uterus by a midline fibrous bundle.
E. the uterine artery runs through the uterosacral ligament (USL) before reaching the uterine body.

308. Total abdominal hysterectomy (TAH) for benign disease:

A. has a higher mortality rate than vaginal hysterectomy.
B. has a 6-week mortality rate of approximately 0.5%.
C. has a sharply rising mortality rate after the age of 40 years.
D. has a postoperative incidence of calf deep vein thrombosis of 3–5% if thromboprophylaxis is not given.
E. requires antibiotic prophylaxis in all cases to reduce infective morbidity.

309. With regard to the appropriateness of hysterectomy for the symptom of heavy periods:

A. a super-plus tampon fully soaked can hold only up to 4 ml of blood.
B. the average blood loss per period is 80 ml.
C. menstrual calendars are significantly more objective than normal history-taking when calculating menstrual blood loss.
D. in the UK the lifetime risk of having a hysterectomy is about 20%.
E. approximately one-third of hysterectomies performed on women below the age of 60 years are on those younger than 40 years.

310. With regard to complications after hysteroscopic surgery for menorrhagia:

A. the most common operative complication is excessive bleeding.
B. perforation of the uterus occurs in about 5% of cases undertaken by experienced operators.
C. complications were audited in the 'VALUE' study of the Royal College of Obstetricians and Gynaecologists (RCOG).
D. the mortality rate from hysteroscopic surgery for menorrhagia is considerably less than that from pregnancy-related causes (maternal mortality) in the UK.
E. septicaemia is a recognized cause of death complicating this type of surgery.

311. In preparation for transcervical resection of the endometrium (TCRE):

A. prior hysteroscopic assessment is generally recommended.
B. drug preparation of the endometrium is generally recommended.
C. large fibroids are generally a contraindication.
D. vaginal ultrasonography is superior to hysteroscopy and laparoscopy in the diagnosis of fibroids.
E. vaginal ultrasonography is superior to hysteroscopy and biopsy in the exclusion of malignancy.

312. Recognized predisposing factors for chronic pelvic pain include:

A. previous chlamydial infection.
B. previous tuberculous endometritis.
C. irritable bowel syndrome.
D. combined oral contraceptive pill.
E. polycystic ovarian syndrome.

313. In women with pelvic endometriosis:

A. menorrhagia is not significantly more common than in age-matched controls.
B. dysmenorrhoea is an almost universal finding on history.
C. deep dyspareunia occurs in about one-third of cases.
D. premenstrual spotting is three or four times more common than in controls.
E. irregularity of the periods is an uncommon feature.

314. In premenstrual syndrome (PMS):

- **A.** symptoms occur at a time of relative progesterone deficiency.
- **B.** more than 90% of women of childbearing age have at least one PMS symptom.
- **C.** 20–30% of cases are not cyclical.
- **D.** response to placebo is very uncommon.
- **E.** gamma-linolenic acid (GLA) is probably the first-choice drug for cyclical mastalgia.

315. With regard to established postmenopausal osteoporosis:

- **A.** oestradiol implants can produce more than a 5% increase in bone density after 1 year.
- **B.** calcium and vitamin D tablets produce no significant benefit.
- **C.** the proximal femur is the most commonly affected site.
- **D.** oestrogen therapy produces increased bone density of both compact and cancellous bone.
- **E.** oestrogen therapy after osteoporotic fracture may prevent further bone loss.

316. With regard to osteoporosis:

- **A.** bone density in the proximal forearm usually correlates well with bone mineral content at other sites.
- **B.** single-photon absorptiometry is the investigation of choice in detecting lumbar spine osteoporosis.
- **C.** bone densitometry uses labelled fluorine as a radiation source.
- **D.** less than 5% of distal forearm bone is trabecular bone.
- **E.** bone loss of 20–30% by the age of 70 years is typical of postmenopausal osteoporosis.

317. With regard to calcium metabolism:

- **A.** a reasonable dietary calcium requirement is 500 mg daily.
- **B.** typical postmenopausal calcium loss in untreated susceptible women is 1 mmol/day.
- **C.** excessive caffeine intake has a deleterious effect on calcium balance in postmenopausal women.
- **D.** the average calcium content of a full-term baby is approximately 150 g.
- **E.** about 45% of circulating calcium is bound to protein.

318. With regard to drugs and osteoporosis:

A. aspirin use in pregnancy can lead to osteoporosis.
B. heparin-induced osteoporosis is prevented by prophylactic fluoride tablets.
C. tibolone use can exacerbate postmenopausal osteoporosis.
D. calcium supplements reduce the rate of bone loss in osteoporosis.
E. tamoxifen protects against osteoporosis.

319. Continuous combined oestrogen and progestogen therapy for postmenopausal women with climacteric symptoms:

A. produces a significant deterioration in the low density lipoprotein/high density lipoprotein (LDL/HDL) ratio.
B. with full compliance can produce a rate of amenorrhoea of 90% or more at 1 year.
C. causes headache as the principal initial troublesome symptom.
D. will have fully prevented bone loss after 5 years of therapy.
E. is more likely to be well tolerated postmenopausally than perimenopausally.

320. Progestogens in hormone replacement therapy (HRT):

A. should be given for at least 12 days per cycle.
B. if given continuously cause fewer side-effects.
C. are usually given at a higher daily dose than the progestogen-only contraceptive pill.
D. reduce HDL concentrations in the plasma.
E. in the form of norethisterone is given in a dose of 5 mg/day.

321. With regard to postmenopausal cyclical combined hormone replacement therapy (HRT):

A. oestrogen is a direct coronary vasodilator.
B. there is an increased incidence of ovarian cancer.
C. 5 years of use will probably halve the mortality rate from ischaemic heart disease.
D. the risk of cerebrovascular accident is significantly reduced after 5 years of use.
E. there is an increased incidence of endometrial cancer.

322. With regard to breast cancer:

A. the overall lifetime risk for all women in the UK is approximately 1 in 12.
B. the risk is approximately doubled after 20 years' HRT use.
C. a history of breast cancer in a first-degree relative increases the risk by 5–10%.
D. previous stage I breast cancer is an absolute contra-indication to HRT.
E. HRT given by implant reduces breast cancer risk.

323. Oestradiol (E_2) levels in postmenopausal women on hormone replacement therapy (HRT):

A. decay more rapidly with reservoir patches than with matrix patches.
B. from a 50-mg patch would usually produce a peak level of around 200–300 pmol/l.
C. will be three to five times higher at the peak with a 50-mg implant than with a 50-mg patch.
D. one 50-mg patch will peak at a level roughly half the oestrogen level at a typical ovulation.
E. are higher with a 50-mg patch than with a 2-mg oestradiol valerate tablet.

324. With regard to lipid levels in women on hormone replacement therapy (HRT):

A. HRT produces a reduction in the level of low density lipoprotein (LDL) cholesterol.
B. the change in the level of LDL cholesterol on HRT is more pronounced with tablets than with patches.
C. HRT produces an increased level of high density lipoprotein (HDL) cholesterol.
D. HRT reduces the concentration of plasma triglycerides.
E. lipid changes confer perhaps 25–50% of the cardiovascular benefit of HRT.

325. Intrauterine adhesions (Asherman's syndrome):

A. may occur following caesarean section.
B. may be due to tuberculous endometritis.
C. is always associated with amenorrhoea or hypomenorrhoea.
D. is associated with normal vaginal bleeding following withdrawal of the combined oral contraceptive pill.
E. is associated with a normal luteal phase serum concentration of progesterone.

326. Expected changes during the perimenopause include:

A. rising follicle-stimulating hormone (FSH) levels.
B. decreasing E_2 levels during ovulatory menstrual cycles.
C. progressive shortening of menstrual cycle length owing to a shorter follicular phase.
D. declining fertility.
E. increasing incidence of luteal phase defects.

327. After the menopause:

A. peripheral conversion of androstenedione is the main source of oestrone (E_1).
B. oestradiol (E_2) is the major oestrogen produced in adipose tissue.
C. osteoporosis is commoner in smokers than in non-smokers.
D. ovarian testosterone secretion increases.
E. circulating androstenedione secretion increases.

328. Concerning fibroids:

A. myomectomy in women with otherwise unexplained infertility results in a pregnancy rate of around 50%.
B. recurrence occurs in 15–30% of cases following myomectomy.
C. preoperative use of gonadotrophin-releasing hormone (GnRH) analogues prevents recurrence following myomectomy.
D. hysterectomy must be performed in a perimenopausal woman with a 12 weeks' size fibroid uterus.
E. may cause postmenopausal bleeding.

329. The following investigations are indicated in a 17-year-old girl with recurrent heavy menstrual loss:
A. thyroid function tests.
B. estimation of serum prolactin levels.
C. pelvic ultrasonography.
D. diagnostic curettage and hysteroscopy.
E. blood picture and clotting screen.

330. During pregnancy, fibroids:
A. have an incidence of 15%.
B. very commonly increase in size.
C. may be associated with preterm labour.
D. could be treated with GnRH analogues.
E. situated at the uterine isthmus are a contraindication to a trial of vaginal delivery after a previous caesarean section.

331. Primary dysmenorrhoea:
A. characteristically starts 2–3 years after menarche.
B. could be treated effectively with the combined oral contraceptive pill in over 80% of cases.
C. could be due to partial obstruction of a uterine horn in a bicornuate uterus.
D. occurs only in ovulatory cycles.
E. could be effectively treated by dilatation of the cervix.

332. Treatment of women with fibroids with gonadotrophin releasing hormone (GnRH) analogues:
A. causes hot flushes in the majority of cases.
B. results in an average decrease of fibroid volume of 75%.
C. produces maximum reduction in fibroid size when the circulating oestradiol level is 150 pg/ml.
D. causes maximum regression of the fibroid uterus size after 12 weeks of therapy.
E. is associated with acute degeneration of fibroids.

333. The following drugs effectively treat uncomplicated genital *Chlamydia trachomatis* infection:
A. nitrofurantoin.
B. erythromycin.
C. flucloxacillin.
D. azithromycin.
E. oxytetracycline.

334. Genital warts:

A. infection may be subclinical, detected only by cytological examination or colposcopy.
B. must be differentiated from epithelial papillae, small sebaceous glands, molluscum contagiosum and neoplastic lesions.
C. are a sexually transmitted disease in most cases.
D. are associated with chlamydial infection.
E. should always be treated.

335. Actinomycosis-like organisms:

A. are harmful when found in the mouth and gastrointestinal tract.
B. in the lower genital tract are detectable only by cytological examination or culture when a foreign body is present.
C. found in a routine smear of coil (IUCD) users appear not to be related to the duration of use of the device.
D. infection throughout the genital tract (frank actinomycosis) is not a serious condition.
E. infection throughout the genital tract (frank actinomycosis) is extremely rare.

336. *Chlamydia trachomatis*:

A. is easily cultured from vaginal discharge.
B. is commonly a cause of vaginal discharge.
C. may be treated with either erythromycin or tetracyclines.
D. can cause neonatal pneumonia.
E. can cause sterile pyuria.

337. Human immunodeficiency virus (HIV) infection:

A. is mainly a problem of homosexual men, worldwide.
B. is more likely to be transferred from a man with HIV to a seronegative woman than from a woman with HIV to a seronegative man.
C. is a problem amongst lesbian women.
D. is caused by a retrovirus.
E. transmission is prevented by the use of the contraceptive diaphragm.

338. Bacterial vaginosis:
- **A.** is the commonest cause of vaginal discharge in women.
- **B.** causes vaginal soreness as its main symptom.
- **C.** may be asymptomatic.
- **D.** is not associated with perioperative gynaecological morbidity.
- **E.** is characterized by a vaginal pH lower than 5.

339. Pelvic inflammatory disease (PID):
- **A.** should be regarded by healthcare professionals as a sexually transmitted disease.
- **B.** is caused mainly by gonorrhoea in the UK.
- **C.** is associated with asymptomatic, non-specific urethritis (NSU) in male partners.
- **D.** does not require contact tracing.
- **E.** may not reveal any pathological organism on culture of swabs from the endocervix or vagina.

340. *Trichomonas vaginalis* (TV) infection:
- **A.** rarely causes severe vulval soreness.
- **B.** may present similarly to bacterial vaginosis.
- **C.** is a sexually transmitted disease.
- **D.** should be treated with multiple drug therapy.
- **E.** is caused by a uniflagellate protozoan.

341. Syphilis:
- **A.** testing is no longer part of antenatal screening in the UK.
- **B.** may be responsible for mid-trimester abortion.
- **C.** is easily distinguishable from yaws, serologically.
- **D.** is curable.
- **E.** infection is an indication to test for HIV.

342. Genital candidiasis:
- **A.** is the commonest cause of vaginal discharge in the UK.
- **B.** is usually initially treated with triazoles.
- **C.** may be resistant to topical and some oral preparations.
- **D.** can cause fissuring of the perineum.
- **E.** is regarded as a sexually transmitted disease.

343. Genital herpes simplex virus (HSV):
- **A.** can be transmitted by oral sex.
- **B.** is caused by a retrovirus.
- **C.** treatment is often to alleviate symptoms.
- **D.** recurrence occurs in about 90% of those who have a primary attack of HSV-2.
- **E.** can cause urinary retention.

344. Clear-cell vaginal cancer following in utero exposure to diethlyl stilboestrol (DES):
- **A.** is more common if exposure occurred in the first trimester.
- **B.** has a peak incidence between 25 and 30 years.
- **C.** should be prevented by performing total vaginectomy in women developing vaginal adenosis.
- **D.** should be prevented by performing total vaginectomy in women developing vaginal intra-epithelial neoplasia (VAIN).
- **E.** has the same age-distribution as in the non-exposed population.

345. Donovan bodies are associated with:
- **A.** syphilis.
- **B.** gonorrhoea.
- **C.** herpes genitalis.
- **D.** *Chlamydia trachomatis* infection.
- **E.** granuloma inguinale.

346. In the presence of an 'ectopy' of the ectocervix, a cell scraping would most likely contain abundant:
- **A.** endocervical cells.
- **B.** lymphocytes.
- **C.** anucleated squamous cells.
- **D.** intermediate cells.
- **E.** histocytes.

347. In the repair of a rectovaginal fistula:

A. a temporary colostomy should always be performed.
B. malignancy should first be excluded.
C. colpocleisis is recommended.
D. a low-residue diet in the postoperative period is recommended.
E. the patient should be warned that there may be some (initial) narrowing of the vagina.

348. Causes of faecal incontinence include:

A. damage to the pudendal nerve.
B. a rectovaginal fistula.
C. a second-degree vaginal tear.
D. a ring pessary.
E. an impacted rectum.

349. The following are suitable for treatment as a day-case:

A. a fit 58-year-old woman who lives alone for a D&C and hysteroscopy.
B. a 24-year-old asthmatic for laparoscopy and dye.
C. a fit 32-year old woman with extensive vulval warts for laser treatment.
D. a fit 18-year-old woman for termination of pregnancy of 16 weeks' gestation.
E. a 24-year-old woman with sickle cell disease for laparoscopic sterilization.

350. Pain at the lateral end of a Pfannenstiel incision may be caused by:

A. the knot of a suture.
B. genitofemoral nerve entrapment.
C. a neuroma.
D. a spigelian hernia.
E. rectus abdominis syndrome.

351. A 38-year-old woman is referred by her GP with a past history of PID and 7 weeks' amenorrhoea associated with slight PV blood loss. Ultrasonography (transabdominal) performed the previous day shows a single intrauterine sac with a mean sac diameter of 16 mm. No fetal parts were visualized. The following statements are correct:

A. The ultrasonographic findings are consistent with an anembryonic pregnancy and urgent dilatation and curettage should be arranged.
B. Repeat ultrasonography should be arranged after 1 week.
C. This is an ectopic pregnancy and urgent laparoscopy is mandatory.
D. Estimation of serum β-human chorionic gonadotrophin (β-hCG) levels and transvaginal ultrasonography should be arranged.
E. Conservative management is appropriate if the β-hCG level falls after 5 days.

352. Septic shock in a gynaecological patient:

A. is characterized by tachycardia and hypotension.
B. does not cause renal failure.
C. results in adult respiratory distress syndrome.
D. will require high-dose opioid treatment.
E. has a high mortality rate.

353. The vagina:

A. develops partially from the urogenital sinus.
B. recanalizes at 20 weeks postconception.
C. may be absent in the presence of ovaries.
D. has a pH of 5 or less in the newborn.
E. may be completely absent in the presence of a uterus.

354. With regard to human sexual differentiation:

A. Müllerian inhibiting factor has a local action.
B. the presence of functioning testes will always lead to a male phenotype.
C. testicular differentiation factor is present on the long arm of the Y chromosome.
D. the presence of functioning ovaries is necessary for the development of female phenotype.
E. oestrogen causes development of the Müllerian system.

355. Increased incidence of venous thrombosis is associated with:
- **A.** abdominal hysterectomy for benign disease.
- **B.** factor V Leiden mutation.
- **C.** use of the progestogen-only pill.
- **D.** ovarian hyperstimulation syndrome.
- **E.** dilatation and curettage.

356. The risk of surgical infection can be reduced by:
- **A.** keeping the theatre doors closed during the operation.
- **B.** careful hand and nail scrubbing with a brush between cases.
- **C.** scheduling the potentially infected cases at the end of the list.
- **D.** the use of natural non-absorbable suture material.
- **E.** routine drainage for all operations.

357. With regard to female sterilization:
- **A.** the failure rate of postpartum sterilization is lower than that for interval procedure.
- **B.** failure may be due to tuboperitoneal fistula.
- **C.** surgical errors account for about 5% of failures.
- **D.** the incidence of ectopic pregnancy within 2 years of sterilization is about 2 per 1000 women sterilized.
- **E.** endometrial resection is a reliable method of sterilization.

358. The following are of value in the diagnosis of gonorrhoea in the female:
- **A.** high vaginal swab.
- **B.** naked-eye examination of vaginal discharge.
- **C.** complement fixation.
- **D.** anal swab.
- **E.** examination of the male partner.

359. Emergency contraception:
- **A.** can be taken, in the form of the Yuzpe method, only up to 48 hours after unprotected sexual intercourse.
- **B.** in the form of the intrauterine contraceptive device (IUCD) can be used up to 5 days after the earliest possible day of ovulation (calculated from shortest menstrual cycle).
- **C.** can be given as 25 Microval tablets within 48 hours of intercourse and repeated 12 hours later if oestrogens are absolutely contraindicated.
- **D.** can be used only twice in any one menstrual cycle.
- **E.** should be advised at whatever day in the cycle there has been unprotected sex.

360. Depot medroxyprogesterone acetate (DMPA) injections:
- **A.** are more reliable as a form of contraception than the combined oral contraceptive pill.
- **B.** have a failure rate of 2 per 100 woman-years.
- **C.** can be given within 3 days of childbirth, without any side-effects.
- **D.** are given every 8 weeks as a routine.
- **E.** do not affect blood pressure.

361. Norplant (subcutaneous progestogen-only implant):
- **A.** consists of five Silastic capsules containing norethisterone.
- **B.** is effective within 24 hours of injection and lasts for 5 years.
- **C.** can cause irregular vaginal bleeding for many months after insertion.
- **D.** has a higher (double) failure rate in women weighing more than 70 kg.
- **E.** removal results in normal fertility only after about 7 days.

362. The copper intrauterine contraceptive device (IUCD):
- **A.** is absolutely contraindicated in a nulliparous patient.
- **B.** should be inserted under antibiotic prophylaxis in the presence of bacterial vaginosis.
- **C.** probably acts mainly by blocking fertilization.
- **D.** should be fitted only during menstruation.
- **E.** leads to a high rate of miscarriage if left in situ with an accidental pregnancy.

363. The female condom:

- **A.** is made from vulcanized latex rubber.
- **B.** is stronger than the male condom.
- **C.** has been found to be acceptable in over 90% of users.
- **D.** must be used with spermicide.
- **E.** theoretically prevents transmission of *Trichomonas vaginalis* infection.

364. Contraception in a girl under 16 years old:

- **A.** should not be given unless parental consent is obtained.
- **B.** should involve the use of condoms as a complementary method only in those at high risk.
- **C.** must be given with full confidentiality to the client.
- **D.** may be provided by general practitioners.
- **E.** is best provided by the intrauterine contraceptive device (IUCD) or condoms.

365. The contraceptive effect of the male condom is reduced if used with:

- **A.** baby oil.
- **B.** Gyno-Daktarin (miconazole) vaginal anticandidal cream.
- **C.** Cyclogest (progesterone) vaginal pessaries.
- **D.** dienoestrol cream.
- **E.** petroleum jelly.

366. The levonorgestrel intrauterine contraception device (IUCD):

- **A.** has a higher ectopic pregnancy rate than the copper IUCD.
- **B.** has a lower failure rate than the copper IUCD.
- **C.** reduces the risk of pelvic infection.
- **D.** may be used in women with climacteric symptoms requiring hormone replacement therapy instead of systemic progestogens to protect the endometrium from hyperplasia.
- **E.** is especially useful in the nulliparous woman.

367. The contraceptive diaphragm:

A. works mainly by acting as a sperm-tight fit across the cervical os.

B. user needs to be comfortable handling her own genitalia.

C. does not need to be used with spermicide.

D. must remain in situ for at least 10 hours after sexual intercourse.

E. may protect the user from cervical neoplasia.

368. When taking the combined oral contraceptive pill:

A. a break in pill-taking is recommended every 5 years.

B. a first migraine is common, unimportant, side-effect in the first 4 months.

C. after childbirth, it should be started at the 6-week postnatal check.

D. condoms should be used for 14 days if a pill is missed by more than 12 hours.

E. extending the 7-day pill-free interval does not increase the failure rate of the method.

369. Absolute contraindications to the combined oral contraceptive pill include:

A. severe thrombotic disease.

B. focal migraine.

C. diabetes mellitus.

D. hypothyroidism.

E. sickle cell disease.

370. The combined oral contraceptive pill:

A. is the commonest method of contraception in the under 30s.

B. in the 'double-Dutch' method is prescribed in association with the male condom.

C. is contraindicated in women with a history of non-focal migraine.

D. cannot be commenced in the middle of the menstrual cycle.

E. is associated with an increase in the risk of venous thromboembolism similar to that during pregnancy.

371. The progestogen-only pill (POP):

A. is contraindicated in a 43-year-old women who smokes ten cigarettes a day.
B. is best taken last thing at night for the lowest failure rate.
C. is associated with a slightly increased risk of ectopic pregnancy.
D. works mainly by inhibition of ovulation.
E. is less contraceptively reliable in the obese woman.

372. Intermenstrual bleeding whilst on the combined oral contraceptive pill:

A. is often referred to as 'breakthrough' bleeding.
B. can be ignored for up to 1 year of use of the combined pill.
C. is usually a sign that the combined pill will not prevent pregnancy in that particular woman.
D. may be caused by *Chlamydia trachomatis* infection.
E. usually indicates the need for a change in method of contraception (i.e. not to use the combined pill any more).

373. The contraceptive effect of the combined oral contraceptive pill is reduced by:

A. carbamazepine.
B. phenobarbitone.
C. phenytoin.
D. sodium valproate.
E. rifampicin.

374. The following conditions are absolute contraindications to taking the combined oral contraceptive pill:

A. age over 40 years.
B. any previous history of migraine with hemianopia.
C. any previous history of trophoblastic disease.
D. otosclerosis.
E. cholestatic jaundice.

375. The following are associated with the use of the progestogen-only contraceptive pill:

A. functional ovarian cysts.
B. acne.
C. arterial thrombosis.
D. increased risk of breast cancer.
E. chloasma.

376. Depo-Provera injectable contraceptive:
- **A.** is associated with virilization of the exposed female fetus.
- **B.** inhibits lactation.
- **C.** may be used in women with a history of thromboembolism.
- **D.** may be used in women with sickle cell anaemia.
- **E.** may be given within 5 days of miscarriage or termination of pregnancy.

377. In England and Wales, if a girl aged under 14 years requests the combined oral contraceptive pill:
- **A.** her parents must be informed.
- **B.** her GP must be informed.
- **C.** she must be accompanied by an adult.
- **D.** she should be warned that taking the pill before attainment of her final height may lead to short stature.
- **E.** this can be prescribed only by a hospital consultant.

378. Intrauterine contraceptive devices (IUCDs) can be fitted:
- **A.** only during the menstrual period.
- **B.** only if the woman is multiparous.
- **C.** as an emergency contraception only if the woman wants long-term contraception.
- **D.** as an emergency contraception only up to 5 days after a single act of unprotected intercourse occurring on day 5 of a regular 28-day cycle.
- **E.** immediately after termination of pregnancy.

379. Symptoms suggestive of detrusor instability include:
- **A.** nocturia.
- **B.** haematuria.
- **C.** being able to interrupt urinary flow.
- **D.** frequency.
- **E.** urgency.

380. The Burch colposuspension:

A. will not correct moderate rectocele.
B. has a long-term incidence of postoperative voiding problems of less than 5%.
C. is relatively contraindicated when the preoperative isometric detrusor pressure is very low.
D. involves suturing the vagina to the retropubic peritoneum.
E. produces more de novo postoperative detrusor instability than vaginal buttressing (anterior repair).

381. In surgery for genuine stress incontinence:

A. the Raz procedure produces 70–80% long-term cure.
B. the Stamey procedure involves plication of the pubo-urethral ligaments.
C. the Marshall-Marchetti-Krantz (MMK) procedure does not involve opening the peritoneum.
D. the Shah endoscopic suspension of bladder neck includes urethrocystoscopy.
E. the Aldridge sling procedure is often performed laparoscopically.

382. Concerning innervation of the bladder and urethra:

A. the parasympathetic supply is from sacral segments S2–S4.
B. the sympathetic innervation is concentrated at the bladder neck.
C. the micturition centre is in the medulla.
D. noradrenaline is the predominant neuromuscular transmitter.
E. normal voiding is effected by sympathetic innervation of the bladder.

383. Female urodynamic investigations:

A. are important in the accurate diagnosis of detrusor instability.
B. normally show a bladder capacity in the range of 300–500 ml.
C. normally show a detrusor pressure on filling cystometry exceeding 15 cmH_2O.
D. in the form of urethral pressure profile are an accurate measurement of urethral function.
E. normally show a bladder voiding flow exceeding 10 ml per second.

384. Colposuspension:

A. may be performed in the presence of cystocele.
B. is a good procedure for controlling uterovaginal prolapse.
C. may exacerbate the development of an enterocele.
D. may be complicated by detrusor instability.
E. may interfere with sexual function.

385. In interstitial cystitis:

A. the patient presents predominantly with urgency.
B. bladder capacity is increased.
C. an infectious cause is often found.
D. mast cell infiltration is seen on bladder biopsy.
E. the best treatment is bladder retraining.

386. Burch colposuspension:

A. should be performed only after urodynamic assessment.
B. is the operation of choice in genuine stress incontinence.
C. is indicated in the absence of vault mobility.
D. may be complicated by detrusor instability after operation.
E. is best managed by means of a postoperative Foley's catheter.

387. Regarding cystourethrometry:

A. an average flow of 15–25 ml per second is normal in females.
B. in bladder hypersensitivity, the pressure rises to above 30 cmH_2O.
C. positional changes in the patient can provoke bladder instability.
D. urethral pressure does not correlate well with urinary incontinence.
E. ambulatory urodynamics are the most reliable method of assessing bladder instability.

388. The following statements are true regarding detrusor instability:

A. Detrusor contractions are seen on cystometry.
B. Patients with uncomplicated detrusor instability have a high flow rate.
C. Cystoscopy is diagnostic in detrusor instability.
D. A midstream specimen of urine (MSU) need not be taken as a part of the investigations for detrusor instability.
E. It is helpful to have a frequency–volume chart filled.

389. In the treatment of stress incontinence:

A. paraurethral injection of collagen is a method of restoring continence by decreasing the urethral resistance.
B. anterior colporrhaphy has a lower success rate for cure of genuine stress incontinence than suprapubic procedures.
C. anterior colporrhaphy can cause less detrusor instability than suprapubic operations.
D. in endoscopic bladder neck suspension operations, such as Stamey's procedure, cystoscopy is carried out only to check elevation of the bladder neck.
E. the Marshall-Marchetti-Krantz procedure will correct a cystocele.

390. The following is true of a Burch colposuspension operation:

A. Before performing a Burch colposuspension it is important to ensure that there is adequate vaginal capacity and mobility.
B. The lateral vaginal fornices can be elevated to each contralateral ileopectineal ligament in a Burch colposuspension.
C. Osteitis pubis is a complication of Burch colposuspension.
D. A Burch colposuspension will not correct a cystocele.
E. A Burch colposuspension will make an enterocele or rectocele worse if present.

391. Sling procedures for stress incontinence:

A. are more commonly used in the presence of a scarred vaginal vault.
B. have a success rate lower than that for the Burch operation.
C. are usually done using desensitized porcine dermis.
D. employ fascia of external oblique aponeurosis.
E. in the form of the Stamey procedure has a good long-term success rate.

392. In the 'dye test' (installation of methylene blue stained saline into the bladder) for urinary fistula:

A. if dye leaks from the cervix, the diagnosis is ureterovaginal fistula.
B. if dye only leaks from the urethral meatus, the diagnosis is stress incontinence.
C. if dye leaks into the vagina, the diagnosis is vesicovaginal fistula.
D. if neither dye nor urine leaks, a fistula has not been demonstrated.
E. if no dye leaks into the vagina but urine still leaks, the diagnosis is ureterovaginal fistula.

393. Vesicovaginal fistula:

A. in the developed world is most commonly caused by obstetric pressure necrosis.
B. in the developing world is most commonly caused by surgery or radiation.
C. should be treated surgically in all cases.
D. repair should be followed by free bladder drainage (catheter) for at least 14 days.
E. is a recognized cause of urinary incontinence.

394. Mifepristone:

A. can lead to nausea and vomiting.
B. is successful in the treatment of ectopic pregnancy in up to 50% of cases.
C. can be used up to 12 weeks' gestation in the UK.
D. leads to fetal abnormalities if used antenatally.
E. may cause skin rash.

395. Regarding the innervation of the female lower urinary tract:

A. afferent fibres from the bladder ascend in the lateral reticulospinal tract.
B. the periurethral muscle is supplied by the pudendal nerve.
C. the external urethral sphincter (rhabdosphincter) is supplied via the pelvic splanchnic nerves.
D. pudendal nerve block causes incontinence.
E. the rhabdosphincter receives a somatic supply from sacral roots S2–S4.

396. Factors predisposing to urinary tract injury during hysterectomy include:
- **A.** congenital anomalies of the genital tract.
- **B.** previous pelvic inflammatory disease.
- **C.** previous caesarean section.
- **D.** crossed ectopia.
- **E.** endometriosis.

397. Factors predisposing to urinary tract infection in the female include:
- **A.** spina bifida.
- **B.** the contraceptive diaphragm.
- **C.** diabetes mellitus.
- **D.** urethral stricture.
- **E.** the combined oral contraceptive pill.

398. Surgical procedures to correct genuine stress urinary incontinence aim to:
- **A.** prevent bladder neck relaxation at voiding.
- **B.** fix the position of the proximal urethra as a pelvic structure.
- **C.** increase the urethral closure pressure.
- **D.** increase the functional urethral length.
- **E.** increase bladder neck support.

399. Features of Turner's syndrome include:
- **A.** kyphoscoliosis.
- **B.** cystic hygroma.
- **C.** cubitus valgus.
- **D.** lymphoedema.
- **E.** coarctation of the aorta.

400. There is an increased risk of thromboembolism in association with:
- **A.** postmenopausal hormone replacement therapy (HRT).
- **B.** the combined oral contraceptive pill containing third-generation progestogens, over and above the risk associated with pills containing older progestogens.
- **C.** pregnancy, over and above the risk associated with combined pill.
- **D.** thrombocytopenia.
- **E.** the progestogen-only pill.

Answers

295. AB

Thromboembolic complications account for about 20% of perioperative deaths following hysterectomy. Low-dose heparin has been shown to be effective in reducing the risk of thromboembolism, but is associated with a 5–15% increase in the incidence of wound haematoma. However, there are no significant changes in postoperative haemoglobin levels or blood transfusion requirements. The risk of haematoma can be minimized by administering the heparin well away from the incision site.

Osteoporosis is a well-recognized risk of prolonged heparin administration, and may result in fractures in about 1 in 50 women receiving prolonged antenatal low-dose heparin. The question, however, relates to prophylaxis in gynaecological surgery where heparin is usually used for only a few days.

296. BE

The incidence of Turner's syndrome is 1 in 10 spontaneous abortions and 1 in 2500 live births, suggesting that about 97% of Turner's syndrome zygotes are aborted spontaneously. Patients with Turner's syndrome are phenotypically female with short stature, normal intelligence, ovarian dysgenesis, neck webbing, increased carrying angle (cubitus valgus), broad chest and widely spaced nipples, low posterior hairline, pigmented naevi, coarctation of the aorta and renal anomalies, especially horseshoe kidney. As a result of ovarian dysfunction, oestrogen levels are decreased and gonadotrophin levels are raised (hypergonadotrophic hypogonadism). The decreased oestrogen levels cause delayed secondary sexual characteristics, primary amenorrhoea and premature menopause.

297. AB

In British law, doctors are required to practise to the standard of the ordinary skilled person professing to have that particular skill. When injury to a patient occurs as a result of the normal risks of a particular procedure, this does not constitute negligence. A retained swab or the absence of informed consent *always* constitutes negligence. A failed sterilization (which has been performed correctly) does not constitute negligence if the patient was counselled about the risks of failure before the operation. A clinical error in not, in itself, evidence of negligence or legal liability, and a frank admission of error and proper explanation to the patient or relatives may prevent a claim: many allegations of negligence arise solely from failure of communication.

298. CDE

There are considerable variations in the rates of D&C between different developed countries; in 1989–1990 there were 71.1 D&C procedures per 10,000 women in England, compared with a rate of 10.8 per 10,000 women in America. These variations strongly suggest that D&C may frequently be used inappropriately. Old indications should be reconsidered to determine their appropriateness.

In women under the age of 40 years with menorrhagia (regular but heavy and/or prolonged menstrual bleeding) D&C is not indicated as a primary investigation because it is unlikely to detect gross pelvic pathology. Less than 5% of cases of endometrial adenocarcinoma occur under the age of 40 years, and D&C should be reserved for cases where there is failure of uterine bleeding to respond to medical treatment or persistent intermenstrual bleeding. Other investigations such as outpatient endometrial sampling, pelvic ultrasonography (particularly with a transvaginal transducer) and hysteroscopy should also be considered. Infertility is not an indication for D&C as modern hormonal serum assays are more accurate and less invasive in determining the hormonal status.

299. ABCD

Candidiasis is a common vaginal infection accounting for 28–37% of cases. It is common in the newly sexually active and in those aged under 25 years. A history of pruritus, dyspareunia and a non-offensive curdy discharge is common.

Careful inspection of the vulva and vagina will confirm the presence of erythema. Microscopy slides prepared with a drop of 10% potassium hydroxide show fungal mycelia, and the pH will be less than 5. Cervical cytology smears may show *Candida* but are not a reliable diagnostic index. Swabs should be sent in transport medium for specific *Candida* culture. For uncomplicated attacks of vaginal candidiasis there are no clinically significant differences in the efficacy between the various licensed types and durations of azole antifungal treatments. Cure rates are in the order of 80–90%. Practical differences include: patients prefer 1-day courses and oral treatment over vaginal treatment. Oral agents may be preferable if inflammation is present as some women experience an irritant reaction to particular vaginal pessaries. Oral treatment is more expensive and may not be safe in pregnancy. Vaginal pessaries may cause condom or diaphragm failure.

300. D

One per cent of women will present more than six times a year with vaginal candidiasis. They are invariably due to *Candida albicans.* Non-albicans species, particularly *Candida glabrata,* may also cause chronic vaginitis. The condition is not sexually transmitted and rarely associated with other sexually transmitted diseases. It is often associated with high oestrogen states. Referral to a specialist centre is preferable. Antibiotics which are active against vaginal flora may precipitate attacks of candidiasis. Reinfection from the anus or rectum or from the male partner is rare, and co-treatment of these sources does not reduce the relapse rate. The modern low-dose (30 μg) pills do not affect the incidence of vaginal candidiasis. Women with iron and/or zinc deficiency do not differ from controls in the incidence of vaginal candidiasis.

301. BCD

Bacterial vaginosis is a clinical syndrome of vaginitis with a grey (85% of cases), homogeneous malodorous discharge with a pH of 5.0–5.5 without yeast forms or trichomonads. It is a polymicrobial condition, predominated by anaerobes, lactobacillae and increased concentration of *Bacteroides* species. The amines produced by these species are responsible for the offensive discharge, which is the presenting feature of this condition. Up to 30–40% of women are asymptomatic and the condition is rarely sexually transmitted.

302. CE

There are three stages in the life of a female in which the vagina is atrophic: before the menarche, during lactation and after the menopause. Most women with postmenopausal vaginal atrophy are asymptomatic and vaginitis is rare. Examination of a vaginal smear is diagnostic, showing large numbers of intermediate and parabasal cells with an absence of mature superficial squamous cells. Local oestrogen is initially poorly absorbed, so treatment should be continued for 4–6 weeks.

303. BCD

DES is a non-steroidal synthetic oestrogen. It was synthesized in the UK in 1938 and became readily available as an inexpensive, potent, orally active oestrogen. Towards the end of the 1940s and during the 1950s, DES was used widely in the USA as a 'pregnancy-preserving' agent to prevent miscarriage. The rationale for its use was based on work showing that it stimulated the placenta to produce increased amounts of both oestrogen and progesterone. Over four million women were treated in the USA. DES achieved a somewhat reserved popularity in the UK where fewer than 15,000 women were treated. Its use stopped abruptly in 1971 when an association was noted between DES in-utero exposure and the development of clear cell carcinoma of the vagina.

Non-malignant or benign epithelial changes are common in DES-exposed females and include columnar epithelium on the cervix and vagina. Transverse vaginal and cervical ridges, which are variously described as collars, rims, cockscombs and pseudopolyps, are reported in about one-quarter of the daughters. Aceto-white epithelium with a medium to fine mosaicism is commonly seen on colposcopic examination. These findings represent metaplasia and should not be treated. Uterine and upper genital tract abnormalities are also common in DES-exposed females. Clear-cell adenocarcinoma of the lower genital tract is rare in females exposed to DES in-utero, with an incidence of 1:1,000.

304. ADE

In vaginal prolapse, the tissues and ligaments are usually weak and so any procedure that leaves an adequate vagina is prone to recurrent prolapse. Small bowel prolapse of the vault (enterocele) is a true hernia with a sac that must be opened and excised. To prevent recurrence, the vagina must be either obliterated (Le Fort's procedure) or fixed up internally, usually to the sacroperiosteum (sacral colpopexy). This procedure may be performed abdominally or via a midline posterior vaginal incision. The Manchester and Fothergill repairs are the same, involving anterior repair and cervical amputation flush with the vagina. Posterior repair may or may not be added.

305. AE

The uterosacral and cardinal (transverse cervical) ligaments are the main supports of the uterus. Although they can be taken separately abdominally, in vaginal surgery for prolapse they tend to be atrophic and are taken as one pedicle. If, however, the cardinal ligaments are very thick it may be necessary to take a cardinal pedicle before opening the posterior peritoneum. Manchester repair preserves the supravaginal part of these ligaments, and is performed instead of vaginal hysterectomy when the ligaments are not too slack. This helps prevent future enterocele or vault prolapse. Ovarian removal is more difficult vaginally as the infundibulopelvic pedicle is sometimes hard to reach. The ovarian ligament is thus usually taken (leaving the ovaries behind).

306. D

LASER is an acronym for Light Amplification by Stimulated Emission of Radiation. Laser surgery became very popular but the popularity is now declining. The equipment is very expensive and is technically more difficult to use than electrical machinery (e.g. diathermy). Compared with loop excision for cervical intraepithelial neoplasia, two visits are required and a poor histological specimen is provided, and there is no real benefit in terms of cure. Laser treatment of VIN has given way to local excision, which is easier to perform and less painful. These advantages do not necessarily apply in the treatment of VAIN, where laser still has a place. NdYAG laser is absorbed by protein and produces 3–5-mm depth of coagulation. It is therefore a good coagulator and evaporator, whereas carbon dioxide laser is absorbed by water, produces a very tiny thickness of coagulation (depending on power and exposure time) and is thus a good scalpel.

307. D

The ovary is connected to the uterus by the ovarian ligament (a remnant of the gubernaculum). In TAH with bilateral salpingo-oophorectomy (BSO), the infundibulopelvic ligaments are cut to release the ovaries. The ureter is found at the base of the posterior leaf of the broad ligament, running parallel to it. It is most commonly damaged at the infundibulopelvic ligament or at the vaginal angle, where it tunnels below the uterine artery. This tunnel is always lateral to the USL, so vault bleeding medial to this can be stitched without risk of ureteric damage. There is a fibrous bundle just below the uterovesical fold of the peritoneum, which often bleeds when pushing the bladder down at TAH.

308. AE

The 6-week mortality rate for TAH in Finland in the late 1980s was about 12 per 10,000 procedures. An earlier Danish study showed a mortality rate of 16 per 10,000. This rises to 83 per 10,000 for women over 60 years old, compared with 28 per 10,000 for vaginal hysterectomy in the same group. In these studies the rates for women aged under 40 years and 40–50 years were much the same (4 per 10,000). The overall figures represent a major reduction over those of the previous two decades, and improved thromboprophylaxis has been particularly important in this respect. Deep venous thrombosis (DVT) classically presents 7–10 days after operation, when the patient may have gone home, and so all but major clinically evident DVTs may have been missed in the past. Certainly one study of fibrinogen uptake studies at 10 days showed DVT rates of up to 20% in subjects not receiving prophylaxis. It is clear that antibiotic prophylaxis also produces an overall benefit when given to all patients.

309. CDE

Calculation of menstrual loss by exact methods is messy and cumbersome. A good history is useful, bearing in mind that a super-plus tampon can hold up to 12–15 ml of blood. Women do not usually leave a tampon to that degree and so may change after perhaps 3–5 ml of loss. Some 20 to 30 such tampons per period would thus constitute borderline menorrhagia, the limit of normal being 80 ml. A menstrual chart is significantly better at collecting such information than a history alone. Referral rates by general practitioners differ by up to 300%, resulting in inappropriate referrals. It is generally reckoned that too many hysterectomies are currently being performed, given that up to 20% of women will eventually have the procedure. One-third of those done before the age of 60 years are in women under 40 years, at a time when actual pathology is less common.

310. E

Hysteroscopic surgery for menorrhagia is considerably less hazardous than conventional surgery. The benefits affect morbidity more than mortality, however. Morbidity is vastly reduced, with most patients being normal within days. However, deaths do occur, particularly – but not exclusively – with inexperienced operators. In the Scottish survey, there was one death from septicaemia in 1000 cases. Antibiotic prophylaxis, therefore, is highly recommended. The most common complication is fluid overload, but the number of deaths from this cause has reduced since stricter guidelines have been better adhered to. Perforation of the uterus is not necessarily serious, but bowel perforation may not be recognized and several deaths have resulted from this. Laparoscopy is therefore needed after uterine perforation. The MISTLETOE (Minimally Invasive Surgical Techniques – Laser, EndoThermal Or Endoresection) survey of the RCOG looked at these procedures but much larger and more long-term studies are needed to obtain a full picture of risks. The VALUE (Vaginal, Abdominal or Laparoscopic Uterine Excision) hysterectomy survey is of short-term complications associated with the different methods of hysterectomy for benign disease. Both these surveys have been coordinated by the Medical Audit Unit of the RCOG. Currently, abdominal hysterectomy for benign disease has a mortality rate of about 0.5–1 per 1000 procedures, which is five to ten times that of pregnancy (10 per 100,000). The mortality rate for hysteroscopic techniques is currently thought to lie somewhere between the two.

311. ABCD

It was previously considered to be mandatory to perform hysteroscopy before TCRE, followed by 1–2 months of drug-induced endometrial atrophy. Most still perform hysteroscopy, but a vaginal scan is better at diagnosing fibroids or a bulky uterus, both being predictors of possible failure. Vaginal scanning is not, however, as good at ensuring suitability for a hysteroscopic procedure, or at excluding cancer. Most surgeons still use a preoperative drug such as danazol or a gonadotrophin-releasing hormone analogue. Some operators now omit this, but presumably have the skill to judge the depth of resection by hysteroscopic appearance, as opposed to cutting to a standard depth.

312. AC

Chronic pelvic pain syndrome (CPPS) is a poorly understood cause for dysmenorrhoea-like pain that is not specifically immediately premenstrual. The pain is typically felt in both groins, the suprapubic region and presacrally. It is characteristically present for an increasing amount of the menstrual cycle until it lasts for 3 weeks or is even continuous. The pain is made worse by sexual intercourse. Sex hormone derangement such as in polycystic ovarian syndrome is not a predisposing factor. The combined oral contraceptive pill might seem a reasonable therapy, as it helps in normal dysmenorrhoea, but clinically has a very limited place. Only laparoscopy will distinguish it from endometriosis, and in CPPS marked venous congestion of the broad ligaments is often seen. The cause is unknown but predisposing factors include previous chlamydial infection and a neurotic personality. Simple analgesia is often ineffective, but anti-inflammatories, antidepressants and continuous progestogens have all been shown to be useful in some patients. Complementary therapies such as acupuncture may work via endorphin release. In severe cases surgery includes venous transection, uterine nerve ablation and hysterectomy, and even presacral neurectomy may very rarely be needed.

313. ACE

The symptoms of endometriosis are not especially related to its severity on laparoscopy. A skewed view is obtained if looking purely at the selected population of women with gynaecological symptoms. A large study from Aberdeen of women having laparoscopy for sterilization or infertility compared symptoms of those with and without endometriosis. Neither menorrhagia nor premenstrual spotting was more common in endometriosis. The characteristic symptoms were pelvic pain (53%), dysmenorrhoea (61%) and deep dyspareunia (30%), all of which were significantly more common than in women with a normal pelvis. However, many women with endometriosis were asymptomatic, and no explanation for this has been forthcoming.

314. BE

More than 90% of women have at least one PMS symptom, and PMS is always cyclical, by definition. PMS symptoms characteristically occur in the premenstrual week and only when ovulation has occurred. This has led to the theory that PMS symptoms may be due to progesterone excess, and certainly the symptoms are similar to those of progestogenic side-effects. However, some have successfully used progestogens to treat PMS. Perhaps this is analogous to a down-regulation. Certainly some hormone replacement therapy users suffer PMS-like symptoms in the progestogen phase, and this is obliterated by taking continuous progestogen. Oil of Evening Primrose contains GLA, which is particularly good for mastalgia, but without the side-effects of danazol. PMS, being a collection of subjective symptoms and psychological complaints, is a very difficult syndrome in which to measure success of therapy. This is made worse by the fact that, unlike other syndromes, placebo actually works in PMS, often producing significant benefit in trials. Suppression of the ovarian cycle is regarded as the ultimate treatment of PMS, and this is usually achieved with the combined oral contraceptive pill.

315. ADE

The principal established therapy for prevention of the usual postmenopausal bone loss is oestrogen replacement therapy (ERT). The normal rate of bone loss is fast initially (e.g. 3% in the first year) and thereafter levels out at a loss of about 1% per year. Cancellous bone (such as the spine) is the principal type affected, but compact bone (as in the long bones) is also lost. ERT not only prevents loss, but actually increases bone density. ERT will also increase bone density in established osteoporosis. Implants give a far higher dosage of ERT than tablets or patches, and so produce more bone gain. If ERT is not tolerated, calcium-vitamin D tablets will have a small but significant benefit in the prevention of bone loss.

316. AE

Single-photon absorptiometry of the proximal forearm is reported to correlate well with bone mineral content at other sites and with total body calcium. ^{125}I is the radiation source. The distal forearm has a trabecular bone content of about 55%, and the proximal forearm about 13%. Dual-energy X-ray absorptiometry (DEXA) scan is more accurate for measuring bone density of the lumbar spine and hip. Bone density can diminish postmenopausally by about 3% in the first year and by as much as 1% or more annually thereafter. In susceptible women, this means 20–30% bone loss by the age of 70 years.

317. ABCE

An average adult female skeleton has a calcium store of about 1000 g. The total calcium content of a term fetus is about 20–30 g. Calcium is also demanded in pregnancy by extracellular fluid expansion, increased renal loss, the (usually) increased calcification of the maternal skeleton and the demands of lactation. Breast milk contains about 0.8 g calcium per litre. During lactation, the maternal bone mineralization of pregnancy reverses and may cause significant bone loss if the diet is depleted of calcium. This applies especially to pigmented skinned races in darker northern countries, where less ultraviolet light gets through to activate vitamin D synthesis. In winter months, women at risk (especially breastfeeding Asian women in the UK), should be on calcium-vitamin D tablets. The Asian diet is often low in calcium. A reasonable dietary intake is 500 mg/day. Calcium loss via the kidneys is increased by excessive sodium or caffeine intake. Normal brisk weight-bearing exercise also protects against osteoporosis, but very vigorous exercise may have the reverse effect, particularly in underweight female athletes with minimal endogenous oestrogen from body fat.

318. E

The use of heparin in a dose of 10,000 units or more per day for 22 weeks can lead to symptomatic osteoporosis; occasionally it can occur at lower dosages. This bone loss is reversible. The cause of the problem is unknown, but it may be that heparin affects circulating vitamin D or mast cells. Despite the usual mineralization of bones during pregnancy, pregnancy-associated osteoporosis is a recognized phenomenon, and is made more likely by prolonged heparin therapy. Oestrogen is not the only drug that protects against osteoporosis: tamoxifen (which has some oestrogenic properties) also does. Tibolone, being something between an anabolic steroid and an oestrogen, should do so but is not yet licensed for osteoporosis prevention in the UK (1996).

319. BDE

Please see the explanation to the following question.

320. ABCD

Progestogen is needed in combined HRT to oppose the proliferative effect of oestrogen on the endometrium, which could lead to hyperplasia or even malignancy. Most endometrium would undergo secretory change with fewer than 12 days' therapy, but only 12 days of minimum progestogen will virtually guarantee secretory change. The usual dose of norethisterone is 1 mg, compared with the progestogen-only pill dose of 350 μg. This dose is sufficient in some women to produce unpleasant progestogenic (cyclical) side-effects. Recent reports suggest that such effects are reduced if the progestogen is given continuously. Some would therefore question the need for a dose as high as 1 mg, when the progestogen-only pill dose is one-third of this. There is, therefore, a current trend to give very low-dose continuous progestogen, particularly in women already past the menopause, which will often produce amenorrhoea, atrophic endometrium and no progestogenic-side effects. The amenorrhoea rate will depend on the amount of circulating endogenous sex hormones. After 2 years beyond the menopause, the rate will be about 95%. Initially, irregular spotting is common, particularly in the first 3 months. This is the principal symptom that discourages compliance – oestrogenic and progestogenic side-effects are unusual. Continuous combined HRT protects fully against bone loss. The dose of progestogen in such therapy does have a minor deleterious effect on HDL (which is lowered) but this is not clinically significant.

321. ACD

Postmenopausal oestrogen replacement appears significantly to reduce mortality from cardiovascular disease. Studies have reported a reduction of 30–70%, which is most marked in women going straight on to HRT from the menopause. This effect is mediated in several ways, including direct coronary vasodilatation and the beneficial effect on plasma lipids. The risk of stroke is also significantly reduced at 5 years. HRT may have a protective effect against ovarian cancer but much less than that of the combined pill.

322. A

Lifetime breast cancer risk is approximately 1 in 12, making it the most common cancer in women. An increased risk is the main fear of prolonged HRT use. Evidence in the past has been conflicting, but meta-analysis suggests a 30–40% increase in risk after 20 years' use. Some recent large studies, however, have implied that the risk may begin to increase as early as 5 years of use. A first-degree relative having had the disease has a significant effect on risk, probably increasing it by more than 50%. Implants give a far higher oestrogen level than other forms of HRT and so, if anything, may increase the breast cancer risk.

323. ABCE

An anovulatory woman in her 40s might expect a tonic oestradiol level of 200–300 pmol/l. This is the level, therefore, at which HRT may reasonably aim. The actual level produced depends not only on the preparation, but also on the woman's physiology, there being a wide range of mean levels for the same preparation. Generally, a 50-mg patch or a 2-mg oestradiol valerate tablet is thought to produce an E_2 level of 200–300 pmol/l. In an individual women, the level would be higher with a patch, as the patch E_2 escapes the first-pass effect on the liver. Oral E_2 is mostly converted to oestrone (E_1), giving a reversal of the normal 2:1 of E_2:E_1 levels (this is not so with the micromized E_2 oral preparation). Implants give a far higher level of E_2 than other forms of HRT, often reading four figures. This is worrying, as tachyphylaxis in some means even higher levels are reached by more frequent implants. These levels should do no harm in the short term, being very similar to ovulatory levels. In the long term, however, breast cancer risk has to be considered.

324. ABCDE

Heart disease is the biggest killer of women, and its incidence is thought to be at least halved by the taking of HRT. This is mediated partly by a direct coronary vasodilatation, partly by unclear effects, and partly (perhaps 25–50%) by changes in lipid metabolism. The lipid risk factors for ischaemic heart disease (IHD) are increased levels of triglycerides and LDL cholesterol, and reduced levels of HDL cholesterol, especially HDL_2. These changes are reversed by HRT in a dose-dependent way. The effect is greater with oral preparations as they pass through the liver before reaching the circulation, and the liver is the site of main control of lipid metabolism. This begs the question as to whether women with cardiovascular risk factors should preferentially be offered oral rather than parenteral HRT.

325. ABE

Factors associated with Asherman's syndrome are curettage of the pregnant or recently pregnant uterus, infection (endometritis) and uterine surgery (myomectomy, caesarean section). Although patients usually present with secondary amenorrhoea or hypomenorrhoea, Asherman's syndrome may exist in those with normal menses. In addition to the patient's history of previous uterine trauma or infection, failure of withdrawal bleeding following sequential oestrogen-progestogen or the combined oral contraceptive pill conforms the diagnosis. The same is true in women presenting with secondary amenorrhoea and evidence of ovulation.

326. ACDE

Plasma FSH levels start to rise progressively at least 10 years premenopausally, despite normal preovulatory E_2 levels during regular ovulatory cycles. This may be due to a decrease in inhibin levels consequent on a declining number of follicles. High FSH levels in the early follicular phase during the perimenopause lead to accelerated follicle growth and a shortened follicular phase. This is associated with various forms of ovulatory dysfunction including luteal phase deficiency.

327. ACD

The postmenopausal ovarian tissue (theca) responds to raised FSH and luteinizing hormone (LH) concentrations by secreting more testosterone from stromal tissues. E_1, the main oestrogen postmenopausally, is derived from peripheral conversion of androstenedione in adipose tissue. The circulating androstenedione level decreases by 50%, with the majority produced by the adrenal gland.

328. ABE

If fibroid is the only cause of infertility, the pregnancy rate following myomectomy is 50–60% and repeat myomectomy is associated with a less favourable rate. Whether or not GnRH analogues are used, fibroids do recur in at least 15–30% of women following myomectomy. In the asymptomatic perimenopausal woman, no treatment is necessary but follow-up of the size of the fibroid is recommended. Although almost all fibroids regress in size postmenopausally, they still can cause postmenopausal bleeding. Preoperative use of GnRH analogues, intraoperative use of uterine vessels tourniquet and local injection of vasopressin are well-established techniques which help to minimize blood loss during myomectomy. Carefully planned midline vertical incision of the anterior wall or the fundus, through which multiple fibroids may be removed, is ideal. Use of monofilamentous semi-synthetic sutures is associated with less tissue reaction and a decreased incidence of postoperative adhesion formation.

329. ABCE

In adolescents, excessive menstrual loss is due to anovulation in about 70% of cases. Therefore, causes of anovulation such as hypothyroidism, hyperprolactinaemia and polycystic ovary syndrome have to be excluded. Pelvic ultrasonography is also useful in the diagnosis of congenital anomalies of the uterus, submucous fibroids, polycystic ovarian syndrome and other pelvic (ovarian) masses that may be associated with excessive menstrual loss. In adolescents, blood picture, coagulation and endocrine profiles may also be used as indicated, because clotting disorders account for up to 20% of cases in this age group. Invasive procedure are hardly ever justified in these patients to make a preliminary diagnosis.

330. C

Although the incidence of fibroids in the female population is about 20%, that in pregnant women is less than 3%. The likelihood of a fibroid causing symptoms (pain) during pregnancy is unrelated to its size. Ultrasonography follow-up studies during pregnancy have shown that the majority (more than 75%) of fibroids do not increase in size; almost all fibroids decrease in size and become softer during the third trimester. The mode of delivery should, therefore, not be influenced by the mere presence and site of fibroids, but by obstetric factors. Although accidental use of GnRH analogues during pregnancy has not been associated with fetal anomalies, these drugs are certainly not approved for use if pregnancy is suspected or diagnosed. Furthermore, they would not have the same effect on fibroids during pregnancy. In the non-pregnant woman they lead to a hypo-oestrogenic state by inhibiting the hypothalamic-pituitary-ovarian access, and thus reduce the oestrogen-dependent growth of fibroids. During pregnancy, on the other hand, the main bulk of circulating oestrogen is produced by the fetoplacental unit, and not the ovary.

331. BD

The typical onset of primary dysmenorrhoea (painful periods for which no organic or psychological cause can be found) is at or shortly after the onset of menarche. Dysmenorrhoea starting 2–3 years postmenarche should arouse the suspicion of secondary dysmenorrhoea. Primary dysmenorrhoea occurs only in ovulatory cycles. The combined contraceptive pill is effective in over 80% of women with primary dysmenorrhoea, mainly because of inhibition of ovulation, but it also lowers prostaglandin levels in menstrual fluid. Calcium channel blockers (e.g. nifedipine) have been used successfully in the treatment of primary dysmenorrhoea. Procedures such as forced dilatation of the cervix or presacral neurectomy are almost never indicated.

332. ADE

Over 90% of women treated with GnRH analogues report hot flushes and up to 50% complain of other menopausal symptoms. On average, a 50% reduction in fibroid volume is expected and this decrease is maximal after 12 weeks of treatment. However, to be effective in reducing fibroid size, the drug should be given in a dose that decrease the circulating oestradiol concentration to about 15 pg/ml.

Rarely, treatment with GnRH analogues in women with submucous fibroids leads to acute degeneration and subsequent haemorrhage 4–10 weeks after initiation of treatment.

333. BDE

Any of the following regimens is an effective routine treatment for uncomplicated *Chlamydia trachomatis* infection: erythromycin 500 mg four times daily for 1 week; azithromycin 1 g in a single dose; or oxytetracycline 500 mg four times daily for 1 week. However, doxycycline 100 mg twice daily for 1 week probably provides the best method for optimal compliance combined with cost-effectiveness.

334. ABCD

Warts are tumours of the epidermis caused by human papillomavirus (HPV). Most genital warts are transmitted by genital contact, but a small proportion may have common skin warts on the labia majora, pubic region and thighs, from autoinoculation from hand warts. About 6% of women with vulval warts have visible condylomatous lesions on the cervix, but about 50% have subclinical wart virus infection detectable only by cytological examination or colposcopy. Genital warts are associated with *Chlamydia* in 18% of cases. Some warts clear spontaneously, but the majority of patients seen in STD clinics prefer to have them treated.

335. BE

Actinomyces-like organisms may be a coincidental finding in the cervical smears of women with an IUCD. These organisms are normally a harmless commensal in the mouth and gastrointestinal tract. In the lower genital tract, they are detected only by cytology or culture when a foreign body is present. The frequency with which routine smears in IUCD users show these organisms appears to relate in a linear fashion to the duration of use of the device. Frank actinomycosis is an extremely rare and serious (potentially fatal) condition.

336. ACDE

Chlamydia trachomatis is rarely cultured from vaginal discharge. It is an intracellular organism, detected mainly by endocervical sampling. It causes a sterile pyuria and can be identified in the urine. It is usually isolated from an endocervical swab in clinical practice. It is treated by erythromycin or tetracycline. It can cause both eye infections and chest infections in neonates, typically at around 10 days of age. *Chlamydia* is often asymptomatic and is not a common cause of vaginal discharge.

337. BD

HIV infection is globally an infection of heterosexuals. However, in the developed world most infection is amongst homosexual men (not lesbians) and intravenous drug abusers. Infected men are more likely to pass the infection to non-infected women than vice versa. Transmission is not prevented by use of the diaphragm, as only the cervix is protected and not the vagina.

338. AC

Bacterial vaginosis is the commonest cause of vaginal discharge, being responsible for approximately 30% of cases. It may be asymptomatic and usually does not cause vaginal soreness. The pH of the vagina is usually greater than 5. The presence of bacterial vaginosis increases the rate of perio-perative infection for obstetric and gynaecological procedures.

339. AE

PID is caused mainly by sexually transmitted organisms, 60% of which are *C. trachomatis* in the developed world. It is associated with a high incidence of sexually transmitted disease in male consorts, both NSU and gonorrhoea. Contract tracing of all partners should, therefore, be performed. In a proportion of patients, no organisms will be cultured. This may be due to the difficulty of culturing mycoplasmas and ureaplasmas, which can cause PID.

340. BC

TV infection is a vaginal sexually transmitted disease. Contact tracing of all partners should be performed. The infection is caused by a multiflagellate protozoan. TV may present as an asymptomatic infection found coincidentally or as a severe excoriation of the vulva, vagina and upper thighs. The first-line treatment is oral metronidazole.

341. BDE

Syphilis is a treponemal infection that is serologically difficult to differentiate from yaws. Women are still tested antenatally for the infection as it is considered to be curable by penicillin. Syphilis is a cause of mid-trimester abortion. The treatment of syphilis may need to be altered in HIV-infected patients and there may be an increased incidence of syphilis in those affected by HIV.

342. CD

Candidiasis is not regarded as an STD. It is the second commonest cause of vaginal discharge (after bacterial vaginosis). It is usually treated initially by topical imidazoles such as clotrimazole. Some strains of *Candida,* such as *C. glabrata,* may be resistant to topical treatment and to fluconazole orally. Itraconazole may need to be used in this case. Vulval candidiasis may cause fissuring of the perineum.

343. ACDE

HSV-1 infection can be transmitted from the mouth to the genital area by oral sex. HSV-1 and HSV-2 cause herpetic vesicles and ulcers which are extremely painful; salt-water bathing and lignocaine gel can be used to alleviate soreness. Oral acyclovir can be given early in the disease to shorten the length of the illness. After a primary attack of HSV-2, 90% will have a recurrence in the first year, but only 50% with HSV-1. Typing may, therefore, be important in counselling.

344. A

Clear-cell vaginal cancer is a rare complication of in utero exposure to DES, with an estimated risk (calculated from birth to the age of 34) of about one for every 1000 women exposed. Those exposed before 12 weeks have a three times higher risk than those given the drug during the 13th week of gestation or later. The peak incidence occurs between 17 and 23 years. At present it is not known whether a secondary rise will occur for patients beyond the fifth or sixth decade when clear cell cancer occurs more frequently in the non-exposed population. There is no increased risk of pre-invasive squamous cell cancer in the exposed population, and therapy for CIN and VAIN should be identical to therapy given to women who are unexposed.

DES exposed daughters should be meticulously examined as soon as possible after the menarche. They rarely need examination under anaesthesia, but should be advised to use tampons three to six months before their first examination to facilitate colposcopic examination. Careful digital examination will exclude any nodular areas that may be suggestive of clear cell adenocarcinoma. Samples for cytology should be taken from the cervix, endocervical canal and all four vaginal walls. After the application of acetic acid, the transformation zone (TZ) should be noted and any colposcopic vascular patterns recorded. The TZ is often striking for not staining with iodine but biopsies are rarely necessary unless there is a suspicion of a carcinoma present or persistent abnormal cytology needing evaluation. Annual follow up is usually acceptable.

345. E

Donovan bodies are intracellular bodies found in macrophages scraped from granuloma inguinale lesions, a tropical venereal infection caused by the organism *Klebsiella granulomatis* (*Donovania granulomatis*).

346. A

The traditional use of the term 'erosion' for the appearance of visible columnar epithelium on the ectocervix has now largely been superseded by the more correct term 'ectopy'. Erosion literally means loss of the surface epithelium, which does not occur in cervical ectopy. This is a normal finding and is more likely to be present when there are high serum levels of oestrogen, such as during pregnancy or the use of the combined oral contraceptive pill. The cells most likely to be found in abundance in a smear from an area of ectopy are mucin-secreting endocervical cells.

347. BDE

The causes of rectovaginal fistula include malignancy, radiation, surgery, obstetric pressure necrosis, trauma and failed repair of a third-degree tear. If the cause is malignancy, this should be diagnosed (e.g. by biopsy) and treated before attempting surgical repair. A temporary colostomy is indicated in a difficult, high rectovaginal fistula but not in a small mobile one. A low-residue diet in the immediate postoperative period is advised to rest the bowel and promote healing. A satisfactory repair necessitates interposing good tissue (levator ani muscle approximation and/or, in the appropriate case, building up the anal sphincter) between the repaired rectal mucosa and the repaired vaginal epithelium. Colpocleisis was at one time performed for some vesicovaginal fistula repairs; it is very rarely performed now.

348. ABE

Rectovaginal fistula is an obvious cause. The majority of women with idiopathic faecal incontinence have some evidence of pudendal neuropathy, often following a difficult delivery. In the elderly or in patients receiving palliative care with morphine derivatives, faecal impaction may be the cause of incontinence, which can be relieved by disimpaction; a digital rectal examination should never be forgotten.

349. B

Patient A should not be booked for day-case surgery unless she is able to find a responsible adult to stay with her the night after surgery. Patient B would be suitable to book as a day-case (unless the asthma is severe) and, provided there are no adverse events, she should be allowed to go home on the same day. Patient C would not be suitable because of the difficulty of providing adequate analgesia at home. Patient D would not be suitable because of the likelihood of postoperative bleeding. Patient E would not be suitable because of the problems with sickling and the need to ensure adequate oxygenation and hydration. It is no good trusting to luck that these things will not happen.

350. ACE

Neuroma formation can occur with the healing of any severed nerve, and is often microscopic. The genitofemoral nerve divides to give a genital branch that crosses the lower part of the external iliac artery and enters the inguinal canal through the internal ring, whereas the femoral branch descends lateral to the external iliac artery and passes behind the inguinal ligament. It is more likely to catch the iliohypogastric nerve. A spigelian hernia comes through the anterior abdominal wall at the lateral border of the rectus abdominis muscle at the level of the arcuate line, and would therefore be superior to the scar. Rectus abdominis syndrome is one of the myofascial pain syndromes, a large group of muscle disorders characterized by the presence of hypersensitive points called 'trigger points' within a muscle, with a syndrome of pain, muscle spasm, tenderness, stiffness, limitation of motion, weakness and occasionally autonomic dysfunction.

351. BDE

An intrauterine sac of this size is consistent with a normal intrauterine gestation of 6+ weeks; transvaginal ultrasonography may identify either a yolk sac or fetal parts. A confident diagnosis of a normal viable intrauterine gestation can be made only by visualizing the fetus and identifying the fetal heart beat. The sac can be considered abnormal if no fetal parts or yolk sac are apparent with a mean sac diameter of 20 mm. Additional abnormal ultrasonographic findings of a failed intrauterine sac are irregularity of the sac, abnormal implantation site, and irregular or thin (less than 2 mm) trophoblastic reaction. However, none of these signs is sufficiently sensitive or specific to diagnose a failed pregnancy on a single scan; repeat scan after 1 week is therefore appropriate. Normal sac growth is greater than 0.6 mm/day. A pseudo sac (decidual cast) is apparent in 10–20% of ectopic pregnancies and should not be mistaken for an intrauterine pregnancy. An adnexal mass is apparent in 67–95% of cases, a gestational sac in 22–71% and a living embryo in 14–28%. A normal ultrasonographic scan does not exclude the diagnosis of ectopic pregnancy. The correlation of β-hCG and transvaginal ultrasonography increases the sensitivity and specificity of ultrasonography. Heterotopic pregnancy must always be considered; the incidence is 1 in 6000–8000 pregnancies.

352. ACE

Septic shock in any patient has a high mortality rate (over 35%) and must be recognized and treated early. Tachycardia and hypotension in the presence of vasodilatation (if the shock were due to blood loss, vasoconstriction would be evident) and pyrexia should alert to the diagnosis. Occasionally such a patient can present with hypothermia. This patient will require referral to an intensive care unit where direct (rather than indirect) measurements of arterial, central venous and pulmonary arterial pressures can be made.

Therapy is definitive (according to the suspected or known causative organism) and supportive (including oxygen, intravenous fluids, vasoactive drugs, improvement of renal blood flow and sometimes mechanical ventilation). Opioid therapy has no specific role.

353. ABCDE

The vagina develops partially from the urogenital sinus and partially from the paramesonephric ducts. The uterus also develops from the paramesonephric duct. Therefore, in cases of congenital malformation, it would be expected that the presence of a uterus is associated with the presence of the upper part of the vagina at least. Nevertheless, malformations are by definition abnormal, and many malformations cannot be explained by normal development.

354. AC

Sexual differentiation depends on the sex chromosomes, gonadal differentiation and end-organ response. In the presence of a Y chromosome (in addition to at least one X chromosome) the indifferent gonads will become testes. The absence of a Y chromosome (in the presence of at least one X chromosome) will lead to gonadal differentiation as ovaries. The testes will produce testosterone and Müllerian inhibitor. Testosterone will cause development of the male (Wolffian) duct system by direct action. The external genitalia, however, cannot respond to testosterone directly, but need it to be converted to dihydrotestosterone by action of 5α-reductase. In cases of 5α-reductase deficiency there will be functioning testes but a female phenotype. The Müllerian inhibitor causes regression of the female (Müllerian) duct system. In the female it is the absence of testes, and hence testosterone and Müllerian inhibitor, that leads to the female phenotype and development of the Müllerian system.

355. ABD

The Confidential Report into Perioperative Deaths has shown that thromboembolic complications account for about 20% of hysterectomy-associated deaths. All major surgical procedures seem to lead to an increased risk of venous thromboembolism, due partly to the associated immobilization and partly to the changes in clotting factors associated with tissue trauma. Minor procedures such as D&C do not lead to such risk.

Activated protein C (APC) is a naturally occurring anticoagulant. A mutation in a gene related to clotting factor V, called the Leiden mutation, is present in 3–5% of the general population and seems to be associated with APC deficiency, thus predisposing to venous thromboembolism. Some 20–50% of patients with deep venous thrombosis (DVT) studied were found to have the Leiden mutation and APC deficiency. This also applied to patients developing DVT while pregnant or taking the combined oral contraceptive pill. Screening for the Leiden mutation before prescribing the combined oral contraceptive pill or at the beginning of pregnancy has been recently suggested. Thromboembolism is a well-recognized complication of ovarian hyperstimulation syndrome, mainly due to the associated intravascular fluid depletion and the changes in clotting factors secondary to high levels of oestrogen.

356. AC

Although the source of infection in gynaecological patients is usually endogenous, it is important to pay attention to the principles of reducing the exposure of the surgical patient to exogenous organisms. Correct ventilation and regular infection surveillance are essential. During surgery, doors should be closed with minimal movement to ensure correct airflow. The operating list should be constructed with infection in mind, leaving potentially infected cases towards the end and cleaning theatre between cases as necessary. Hand and nail scrubbing with a brush should be meticulous at the beginning of the operation to remove transient flora but further scrubbing between cases is unnecessary. The operation should be handled efficiently with minimal tissue handling and trauma. Haemostasis should be meticulous and consideration should be given to drainage of dead spaces, e.g. cave of Retzius. Routine drainage for straightforward cases is unnecessary. Catgut tends to produce inflammatory reaction and is said to encourage infection at the suture lines, although it is not clear whether or not catgut actually increases the risk of significant postoperative infection.

357. BD

The failure of postpartum sterilization relative to that of interval sterilization varies but may be up to three times higher. Fistula into the peritoneal cavity may develop, allowing the sperm and ovum to meet. This outcome may be facilitated when hydrotubation is performed, either at the time of laparoscopic sterilization or to obtain a hysterosalpingogram afterwards, and is generally inadvisable. Surgical errors, according to most studies, account for 30–50% of failures. The incidence of ectopic pregnancy within 2 years of sterilization is 2 per 1000 women sterilized. A substantial proportion of the failures that do occur will be ectopic pregnancies, and the proportion ranges from 40 to 64%. The risk of ectopic pregnancy does not change with passage of time, whereas the rate of intrauterine pregnancy diminishes. Endometrial resection may act as an effective method of sterilization but there is no adequate information on this yet. Incomplete destruction of the endometrium occurs in many cases and it is not clear whether the tubes are occluded in the process of resection.

358. C

Gonorrhoea is a highly infectious disease that predominantly affects mucosal and glandular structures in the genital tract. A high vaginal swab is not adequate for diagnosis and swabs should be taken from the endocervix, orifices of Bartholin glands and the urethral meatus after milking down of secretion. Microscopic (not naked-eye) examination of a stained smear usually identifies gonococci. Serological tests are usually restricted to epidemiological screening and to women who have already commenced treatment.

359. BCE

The most widely used emergency hormonal preparation is a combined oestrogen-progestogen preparation, the so-called Yuzpe method. The dose taken is two tablets, each containing 50 μg ethinyloestradiol plus 500 μg norgestrel. This is taken as soon as possible after intercourse and not later than 72 hours from the first episode of unprotected intercourse in that cycle. Two further tablets are taken 12 hours later. There is no limit to the number of doses per menstrual cycle, although regular contraception is to be encouraged. Women who cannot take oestrogens (absolute contraindications are history of deep venous thrombosis and focal migraine at presentation) can be given 0.75 mg levonorgestrel (equivalent to 25 tablets of

Microval) taken twice, 12 hours apart, and initiated within 48 hours of intercourse. Efficacy is similar to the Yuzpe method. However, this method is not yet licensed for use. Emergency contraception should be advised at all times of the menstrual cycle when unprotected sexual intercourse has taken place. An IUCD can be fitted following unprotected intercourse up to 5 days after the earliest possible date of ovulation.

360. AE

DMPA is a high-dose progestogen. An intramuscular injection of 150 mg is given every 12 weeks. It acts by inhibiting ovulation with the result that the efficacy of this contraceptive approaches 100%. Almost every drug has side-effects, and DMPA is no exception. Early administration to postpartum women, both breastfeeding and non-breastfeeding, is associated with an increase in menstrual irregularity which can be very troublesome. DMPA does not affect blood pressure.

361. BC

Norplant is a subcutaneous implant consisting of six Silastic capsules containing levonorgestrel. It is effective within 24 hours of insertion and lasts for 5 years. One study, with a different polymer, demonstrated a higher failure rate in women over 70 kg, but the current Norplant is very effective and heavier women do not seem to have a significantly higher failure rate. Some women may have irregular bleeding with Norplant for up to 1 year after insertion. Fertility is restored within a couple of days of removal.

362. BCE

The copper IUCD is now believed to work mainly by the blocking of fertilization. The inflammatory cells of the fluid in the whole genital tract (including the tubes) probably hinder sperm transport and fertilization. The IUCD is not the first choice for the nulliparous patient because of the risk to fertility from infection, especially in those with multiple partners. Several studies have shown that it is possible to insert an IUCD at any time of the cycle, as long as the woman is not likely to have an implanted pregnancy. There is evidence that removal of a copper IUCD in the early part of pregnancy reduces the spontaneous abortion rate from 54% to 20%.

363. BE

The female condom (Femidom) is made from polyurethane and is preloaded with an efficient silicone lubricant. The Femidom has been shown to be less likely to rupture during use. Among 106 volunteers who took part in one of the original studies, more than half found it unacceptable to use. However, the Femidom is expected to protect from sexually transmitted diseases, including *T. vaginalis* infection.

364. CD

A modern low-dose lipid-friendly combined pill usually provides the most suitable method of contraception for under-16s. Injectables are preferable to the IUCD because of their protective effect against pelvic infection. Condoms should always be recommended with the above methods for protection against infection. It is recommended that the girl be encouraged to discuss contraception with her parents, but this is not mandatory before prescription of a method. At all times the young person must have 100% assurance of confidentiality; this is UK law.

365. ABCDE

Vegetable and mineral oil-based lubricants and the bases for many vaginal products that are prescribed will damage rubber used in the male condom. Water-based products such as K-Y Jelly are safe to use. Common products unsafe for use with the male condom are baby oil, Cyclogest, Ecostatin, Gyno-Daktarin, Ortho Dienoestrol, petroleum jelly, Premarin cream and Sultrin.

366. BCD

Studies of the levonorgestrel IUCD have shown it to be highly effective (failure rate of only 0.1–0.3 per 100 woman-years), with an extremely low ectopic pregnancy rate (lower than in women using no method). It also appears to reduce the risk of pelvic infection. However, the inserter has a relatively wide diameter of 4.5 mm, which might make it more difficult to fit in the nulliparous woman. One of the other disadvantages is that the device may cause vaginal spotting for the first few months of use.

367. BE

The contraceptive diaphragm acts mainly as a carrier of the spermicide to the external cervical os and holds the sperm away from the cervical mucus as a barrier. A sperm-tight fit across the true cervix is not possible due to ballooning of the vagina during intercourse. The diaphragm should always be used with spermicidal cream or jelly and should remain in situ for 6 hours after intercourse. It is essential that the user be comfortable with handling her own genitalia and can check the cervix is covered by the diaphragm each time. There is some evidence that women using the diaphragm have a lower incidence of cervical neoplasia.

368. All false

Breaks in pill-taking are not recommended and increase the risk of unwanted pregnancy. A first migraine on commencing the oral contraceptive pill is an absolute contraindication to continuing with the method. The combined pill should be commenced on day 21 after childbirth, as this is when the earliest ovulation has been shown to occur. It should not be used in the breastfeeding woman. Condoms (or other barrier methods, or abstinence) should be used for 7 days after a missed pill (by more than 12 hours). Any missed pill that extends the pill-free interval by more than 7 days increases the failure rate. If the missed pill was the one preceding the pill-free interval, the woman should be advised to start a new packet and miss the normal 7-day break. If, on the other hand, the missed pill was the one following the pill-free interval, she should commence pill-taking immediately and emergency contraception should be used if necessary.

369. AB

Absolute contraindications to the combined contraceptive pill are: severe thrombotic disease, focal migraine, severe migraine requiring sumatriptan ergot, active liver disease, carcinoma of the breast, undiagnosed genital tract bleeding, previous first migraine on the combined pill, systemic lupus erythematosus and pulmonary hypertension. Relative contraindications are: strong family history of ischaemic heart disease, hyperlipidaemia, heavy smoking, diabetes mellitus, gross obesity, sickle cell disease, malignant melanoma, raised blood pressure and oligomenorrhoea (uninvestigated). These are not exhaustive lists but only guidelines.

370. AB

The combined oral contraceptive pill is the commonest method of contraception in the under 30s, sterilization being the commonest in the over 30s. The 'double-Dutch' method of contraception was pioneered in Holland, and is aimed particularly at young people who are at high risk of both pregnancy and sexually transmitted disease. The woman who has had previous migraine not requiring ergotamine or sumatriptan can take the combined pill. The combined pill can be commenced at any time during the menstrual cycle, as long as the woman is not pregnant and understands the need for extra precautions for the first 7 days of pill-taking. It is usually advised that the woman should commence the first packet on the first day of her next period, at which time she does not need to use any other contraception. The risk of venous thromboembolism in women taking the combined pill is between 15 and 30 in 100,000 women each year, compared with 60 in 100,000 pregnant women each year. The background risk for women not pregnant or on the combined pill is 5 per 100,000 per year.

371. CE

The POP can be used in older women who smoke cigarettes. Progestogens do decrease contractility of the fallopian tubes. In POP 'breakthrough' pregnancies, the relative frequency of ectopic pregnancy is increased. The POP acts mainly by its effect on cervical mucus, but a good proportion of users will also not ovulate (this is not its main mode of action). There is a higher pregnancy rate in women weighing over 70 kg. Maximal effect on the mucus is achieved at 4 hours after taking the POP. In some women, the effect on mucus is likely to be at its lowest 14 hours after pill-taking. It is, therefore, best to take the POP approximately 4 hours before the likely time of sexual intercourse.

372. AD

Breakthrough bleeding is common during the first 3 months of commencing a new formulation of the combined oral contraceptive pill. After that time, it should be investigated and/or a new pill chosen. Breakthrough bleeding as a new symptom should be investigated; the main causes are cervical disease, disorder of pregnancy, missed pills, enzyme-inducing drugs and disturbance of absorption. Do not forget *Chlamydia trachomatis* infection causing endometritis and breakthrough bleeding. If all these have been excluded, the woman may need a higher-dose oestrogen pill.

373. ABCE

Drugs that are enzyme inducers lead to increased activity of specific enzyme systems. Other drugs metabolized by the same enzymes will be eliminated more quickly and their therapeutic effect will be reduced. Some antiepileptic drugs are microsomal liver enzyme inducers and lead to increased metabolism of both oestrogen and progesterone, thereby reducing the blood concentration of the combined oral contraceptive pill and the progestogen-only pill by up to 50%. Women on antiepileptic drugs who wish to take the combined pill should be started on a preparation containing 50 μg oestrogen. To ensure that ovulation is inhibited, the serum progesterone concentration should be measured on day 21 of the first cycle on the combined pill (while concomitantly using a barrier method). The progestogens in the pill do not interfere with this assay. If ovulation is not inhibited, the dose should be increased to a dose containing 60 μg oestrogen (two tablets of a 30-μg preparation), and if necessary to 80 μg (30 μg plus 50 μg). Because of the increased drug metabolism, the incidence of side-effects with these higher doses is similar to that associated with the 30-μg preparations. Women on the progestogen-only pill should take double the usual dose. Women on parenteral progestogens (Depo-Provera) are already on a sufficiently high dose and do not need any additional measures. Rifampicin is an antibiotic that is also an enzyme inducer. The antiepileptic drug sodium valproate is not an enzyme inducer.

374. BDE

Women with no other risk factors may continue to take that combined pill up to the menopause. Migraine with hemianopia is a type of 'focal migraine', indicating that cerebral ischaemia is occurring during the attack. The risk of cerebral thrombosis is, therefore, increased and the combined pill could exacerbate this risk. The combined pill may be given after treatment of trophoblastic disease, once human chorionic gonadotrophin levels are undetectable, usually about

2 months after evacuation of hydatidiform mole. Otosclerosis and cholestatic jaundice are adversely affected by pregnancy, and the combined pill may have a similar effect.

375. ABE

Functional ovarian cysts have been shown by ultrasonography to occur in about 50% of women who use the progestogen-only pill (and about 20% of controls). They seldom cause symptoms or require treatment, but the complaint of unilateral pain, with a tender adnexal mass and menstrual irregularity, may mimic an ectopic pregnancy.

376. CDE

No significant fetal abnormalities have been associated with Depo-Provera inadvertently given during pregnancy. Lactating women can use Depo-Provera without adversely affecting lactation. Women with sickle cell anaemia can safely use Depo-Provera; in fact, its use is occasionally associated with a reduction in the frequency and severity of sickling crises.

377. All answers are false

The Law Lords' ruling on the Gillick case (1985) stated that a doctor may prescribe contraception for an under-age girl provided that: (a) the girl is capable of understanding the advice given; (b) the doctor cannot persuade her to inform her parents or allow them to be informed; (c) the girl is very likely to begin or to continue having sexual intercourse, with or without treatment; (d) unless she receives contraceptive advice or treatment, her physical or mental health or both is likely to suffer; and (e) her best interests require contraceptive advice, treatment or both without parental consent. Whether or not contraception is prescribed, the young person is entitled to confidentiality, which should be broken only in the most unusual circumstances, after warning her that this is going to be done and when the doctor is convinced that disclosure can be justified as being in the girl's best interests.

378. E

Many iatrogenic pregnancies are caused by adherence to the myth that it is best to insert the IUCD only during or just after the menses. Not infrequently, the woman who is told to return for fitting with her next period becomes pregnant before the period has arrived. Another cause of 'iatrogenic pregnancy' is removal of the IUCD in mid-cycle, before a new method of contraception has been started, producing the reverse effect of postcoital IUCD fitting. While many women are now aware of the 'morning-after pill', few know that the IUCD can be used as a postcoital contraceptive, or that it can be fitted up to 5 days after the calculated date of ovulation even if this is more than 5 days after intercourse. It is perhaps understandable that GPs and clinics do not take more active steps to promote use of this method, as IUCD fitting is time consuming and requires frequent experience to maintain expertise, but it remains an underused tool in the prevention of unplanned pregnancy. IUCDs are seldom the first-choice method for nulliparous women, as they give no protection against sexually transmitted disease and, if severe PID occurs, future fertility may be jeopardized. Fitting tends to be more difficult for the doctor and more painful for the woman, especially as Nova-T devices are often too long and too wide for the nulliparous uterus, and Multiload products are more traumatic to fit and remove. However, if the woman is unsuitable for the combined pill or Depo-Provera, and the couple is already committed to using condoms as well as a female method, the IUCD has much to recommend it.

379. ADE

Where the patient's sole symptom is stress incontinence, there is an almost 90% chance that this is due to uncomplicated urethral sphincter incompetence (the so-called 'genuine stress incontinence'). Urodynamic investigations are indicated when there are symptoms suggestive of detrusor instability. These symptoms include urgency and urge incontinence; frequency and nocturia; a large amount of urinary loss when incontinent; and inability to interrupt urinary flow. Other indications of urodynamic investigations include adult enuresis, failed previous surgery and abnormal neurological signs. Haematuria is an indication for cystoscopy.

380. ACE

The Burch colposuspension is now established as the most successful procedure in treating genuine stress incontinence. It has short-term success in excess of 90% but, unlike most other procedures, the 5- and 10-year cure rates remain very good. The procedure involves suturing the vaginal angles to the pectineal ligament. This produces a tight support at the bladder neck and explains the main unwanted effect – voiding problems. The incidence of these may be as high as 20% in the long term, particularly if the preoperative isometric detrusor pressure was low. The other main problem of Burch colposuspension is worsening, or even *de novo* development, of any detrusor instability.

381. CD

The Raz procedure produces a good early cure rate, which falls off rapidly with time, being only 50% or less after 5 years; it plicates then elevates the pubourethral ligaments. The Stamey procedure elevates without plication, using a small piece of material such as a piece of arterial graft over the suture to stop it cutting out. The MMK procedure is similar to the Burch colposuspension, but involves sewing the vagina to the posterior pubic peritoneum. The Shah procedure is similar to that of Stamey, but with a different needle, and is called endoscopic, as the bladder neck position is checked urethroscopically. The Aldridge sling is an abdominal procedure, usually performed as a last attempt after previous failed surgery.

382. AB

Innervation of the bladder and urethra is not fully understood. It is supplied by sympathetic, parasympathetic and visceral nerves. The parasympathetic innervation is S2–S4, which run in the pelvic splanchnic nerves. Sympathetic supply is via the superior hypogastric plexus from the thoracic and lumbar segments T10–L2. This is concentrated in the bladder neck. Cerebral control of micturition is complex but appears to be controlled by the pontine centre. The predominant neuromuscular transmitter is acetylcholine. Normal voiding is initiated by the action of parasympathetic nerves.

383. ABE

The bladder is an unreliable witness and therefore urodynamic assessment is mandatory in the accurate diagnosis of urinary incontinence when there are symptoms suggestive of detrusor instability, such as frequency and nocturia. Bladder capacity varies with age, sex and other factors, the normal range being between 300 and 500 ml. The bladder is a low-pressure high-volume system and filling pressures should not exceed 15 cmH_2O on normal filling. Urethral pressure profiles are disappointingly inaccurate in measuring urethral function but may provide some guidance when stress incontinence is not demonstrated clinically. Bladder voiding in females should be assessed carefully because a flow rate of less than 10 ml per second is a contraindication to incontinence surgery.

384. ACDE

Colposuspension will correct a cystocele, although it is ineffective in correcting uterovaginal prolapse and may exacerbate an enterocele. Detrusor instability can be a troublesome problem after operation, occurring in at least 5% of cases, even in the presence of a bladder that was stable before operation.

385. ACDE

Interstitial cystitis is an uncommon cause of the urge syndrome. Urodynamic investigations are normal but the bladder capacity is reduced, which is suggestive of hypersensitivity. The aetiology is unknown but an autoimmune basis is suspected because the levels of complement factors are often raised. Confirmation is by biopsy when mast cell infiltration is seen in association with ulceration of the bladder mucosa. Treatment is fraught with disappointments, and bladder training offers the best outcome.

386. ABD

Operations for urinary incontinence should not be performed without previous urodynamic assessment. The operation of choice is a Burch colposuspension but this should be performed in presence of a reasonably mobile vault. Detrusor instability can be a troublesome problem after operation, even in the presence of a stable bladder before operation (at least 5% of cases). The establishment of normal postoperative voiding is facilitated by the use of a suprapubic catheter.

387. ACDE

Cystourethrometry is generally regarded as an important technique in assessing bladder function and is deemed mandatory before embarking on surgery. Flowmetry is important in assessing urinary flow in women before embarking on procedures that could have an obstructive effect. An average normal flow rate is 15–25 ml per second. In bladder hypersensitivity, the pressure does not rise above 15 cmH_2O despite severe urgency symptoms in the patient, usually resulting in the abandonment of testing. Postural changes can provoke bladder instability. Urethral pressure profilometry is losing favour because pressures do not correlate well with incontinence. Clinical stress is more important than sometimes spurious urodynamic results, especially using the Brown-Wickham technique. Ambulatory urodynamic testing is likely to become the standard technique most likely to elicit detrusor instability.

388. ABE

Cystoscopy is not diagnostic of detrusor instability and is not a helpful investigation but may exclude other bladder pathology like calculi or tumours. An MSU must be sent in all cases of incontinence as an infection may be the cause of urinary symptoms. In addition, it must be done before urodynamic studies because the latter are invasive and may exacerbate an infection. Frequency-volume charts must be filled to evaluate the fluid intake and voiding pattern. The treatment of detrusor instability is almost always conservative, with bladder habit training being the most effective therapy. Anticholinergic drugs such as oxybutynin are useful and imipramine may be used for troublesome nocturia. Cystodistension may produce temporary relief as well as allowing cystoscopy to rule out intravesical pathology.

389. BC

Paraurethral injection of collagen is a method of restoring continence by increasing and not decreasing urethral resistance. In endoscopic bladder neck suspension operations it is essential to perform cystoscopy on all patients after the procedure is completed to ensure that no sutures have passed through the bladder and that the sutures are at the level of the bladder neck. The Marshall-Marchetti-Krantz procedure will not correct a cystocele. A Burch colposuspension will often correct a cystocele.

390. AE

In a Burch colposuspension the lateral vaginal fornices can be elevated towards each ipsilateral ileopectineal ligament thereby elevating the bladder neck. Osteitis pubis is a complication of Marshall-Marchetti-Krantz procedure (0.5–5%) because the sutures are inserted between the paraurethral tissue and the perichondrium of the symphysis pubis. A Burch colposuspension will correct a cystocele. Colposuspension is one of the many procedures being advocated by laparoscopic surgery. It can be approached transperitoneally or extraperitoneally. Comparison with the open Burch procedure is difficult because long-term results have not yet been established for the new procedure. Until a true comparison can be established, the laparoscopic approach will not replace the open procedure. The operation should be used in suitable patients, preferably those who have had no previous incontinence surgery.

391. ABD

Sling procedures are more commonly used as a second-line procedure when scarring has reduced vaginal mobility. Because of this it has a lower overall success rate than a Burch procedure. Although porcine dermis can be used, fascial drugs are more commonly employed. They are normally taken from external oblique aponeurosis but rectus sheath can also be employed. The Stamey procedure, which is technically easier and quicker to perform, has a good short-term success rate but long-term results are poor.

392. BCDE

The dye test is useful in the diagnosis of vesicovaginal fistula. Intravenous pyelography should also be performed to provide information on the function of both kidneys and also assist in the detection of an unsuspected ureterovaginal fistula. Dye leaking through the cervix indicates a vesicocervicovaginal or a vesicouterovaginal fistula. Where there is a ureterovaginal fistula, the dye test would be negative. Always think of the possibility of the rare case where both ureterovaginal and vesicovaginal fistulae are present in the same patient.

393. DE

The main causes of vesicovaginal fistula in the developing world is pressure necrosis from obstructed labour. In the developed world the main causes are surgery, malignancy, radiotherapy or a combination of these; infection also plays a role. It is important to remember that women with vesico-vaginal fistula following, say, abdominal hysterectomy, may present with the complaint of urinary incontinence. Some of these fistulae may heal after prolonged continuous bladder drainage (up to 12 weeks). The basics in surgical repair of these fistulae involve preoperative assessment to confirm the diagnosis and identify the structures involved and the exact location of the fistula. The repair is effected without tension, which necessitates good access and mobilization to approximate good tissues; non-viable or scarred tissue is excised. After operation there should be continuous catheter drainage for 12–14 days.

394. AE

Mifepristone is a progesterone antagonist used for the medical termination of intrauterine pregnancy. It is licensed in the UK for use up to 63 days from the date of the last menstrual period. It is given as a single oral dose of 600 mg, followed 36–48 hours later by a vaginal pessary, 1 mg gemeprost.

395. BCE

Afferent fibres carrying proprioceptive and enteroceptive sensation from the bladder are mediated via sacral roots S2–S4 and ascend in the spinothalamic tracts.

396. ABCDE

Damage to the urinary tract results from the close anatomical proximity between the pelvic organs and the lower urinary tract structures. Such damage probably occurs in about 0.5–1% of all pelvic operations, rising to 2% with radical hysterectomy. The bladder is far more commonly injured than the ureters. Preoperative management directed at prevention of urinary tract injury includes history to elicit predisposing factors. These include previous pelvic inflammatory disease, urinary surgery, irradiation and severe endometriosis which may lead to adhesions and dense scarring, thus altering the pelvic anatomy. The pelvic anatomy may be also altered by a large adnexal mass or broad ligament fibroid.

Congenital anomalies of the genital organs are often associated with congenital urinary tract anomalies, which increase the possibility of injury as a result of the unpredictable variations in the normal anatomy. Duplex ureters occur in about

1 in 125 subjects, most commonly in females, and are bilateral in 1 in 6 cases. A kidney may be absent in 1 in 1100, ectopic in 1 in 900, situated in the pelvis in 1 in 2100, and both solitary and ectopic in 1 in 22,000. Crossed ectopia, taking the ureter in a grossly abnormal path across the pelvis, occurs in 1 in 2000. A history of recurrent urinary tract infection or Müllerian anomalies suggests the need for preoperative intravenous pyelography. Previous caesarean section is the commonest factor predisposing to bladder injury at hysterectomy.

397. ABCD

Infection is the urinary tract disorder most often encountered in a gynaecological patient. Most women experience at least one such infection in the course of their lifetime, and 20% have more than one episode. Most community-acquired infections are due to *Escherichia coli* or, to a lesser extent, *Enterobacter aerogenes*. Hospital-acquired infections, on the other hand, are caused by *Proteus mirabilis* and *Pseudomonas aeruginosa* after catheterization or other bladder instrumentation. Predisposing factors include postmenopausal atrophy, conditions causing incomplete bladder-emptying (e.g. meatal stenosis or urethral stricture), conditions necessitating frequent catheterization (such as spina bifida), bladder stones and diabetes mellitus.

398. CDE

Continence in the female is achieved because the urethrovesical junction and proximal urethra are above the pelvic floor muscles and, therefore, intra-abdominal structures. Any rise in intra-abdominal pressure is transmitted equally to the bladder and proximal urethra, which preserves the pressure gradient and maintains the positive urethral closure pressure. When there is alteration in the bladder neck position, making the proximal urethra a pelvic organ, genuine stress incontinence will result. This is because the rise in intra-abdominal pressure will increase intravesical but not intraurethral pressure. The former will exceed the latter, leading to a negative urethral closure pressure and loss of urine. Surgery aims to restore the intra-abdominal position of the proximal urethra. Bladder neck relaxation occurs during normal voiding and, when demonstrated in urodynamic investigations, is not diagnostic of genuine stress incontinence.

399. ABCDE

Defects in skeletal development include impaired and disordered longitudinal growth, hypoplasia of one or more of the cervical vertebrae and abnormal bone matrix deposition. A key event in the development of the lymphatic system is the establishment of a communication between the jugular lymph sac and the internal jugular vein. This event usually occurs between the fifth and sixth week of gestation. Fetuses with Turner's syndrome usually present a generalized developmental delay. This impairs the formation of lymphatic channels and leads to lymphoedema in many areas. Involvement of the posterior neck area produces the characteristic cystic hygroma. With resorption of the lymphoedema and scarring, webbing of the neck results. Lymphoedema involving the hands and legs often persists until birth. Left-sided cardiac developmental anomalies are particularly frequent. Coarctation of the aorta may be linked to delayed development of the lymphatic system with encroachment on the developing aortic arch.

400. ABC

Despite earlier lack of evidence of an increased risk of thromboembolism in association with hormone replacement therapy (HRT), three epidemiological studies published in 1996 showed a consistent picture of a two- to four-fold increase. The absolute risk in current users (i.e. after subtraction of the background risk) is small, with an estimate in two studies of 16 and 23 excess cases per 100,000 women per year for all venous thromboembolisms, and in a third study of 6 excess cases per 100,000 women per year for pulmonary embolism. The mortality rate from venous thromboembolism is generally about 1–2%. All three studies indicate that the risk of thromboembolism disappears after HRT is stopped. There appears to be no evidence of important differences between types or preparations of HRT.

Recent epidemiological evidence has also indicated that combined contraceptive pills containing third-generation progestogens (gestodene and desogestrel) are associated with a twofold increase in the risk of venous thromboembolism over and above that associated with pills containing older progestogens. The background risk for non-pill users is about 5 per 100,000 women per year, for older pill users 15, for third-generation pill users 30, and for pregnant women 60 per 100,000 women per year. However, the third-generation pill users seemed to have a lower risk of cerebrovascular accident.

Appendix

Detailed Instructions and Sample Answer Sheet for the Multiple Choice Question Papers in the Part 2 MRCOG Examination

The following instructions have been reproduced with kind permission of Mr Roger Jackson, Examination Secretary, Royal College of Obstetricians and Gynaecologists.

Royal College of Obstetricians and Gynaecologists
27 SUSSEX PLACE, REGENT'S PARK, LONDON NW1 4RG
Telephone 0171-262 5425
0171-402 2317

Part 2 Membership Examination Detailed Instructions for the Multiple Choice Question Paper in Obstetrics and Gynaecology

This information must be read very carefully. Failure to follow the instructions will result in failure in the examination.

OFFICIAL COLLEGE IDENTIFICATION CARDS
You will have been issued with an identification card which includes your photograph and College registration number. This will be inspected by the invigilators at the commencement of the examination. If you have lost your identification card or not already received one, you must notify the College immediately. Candidates failing to produce their official College identification card must provide alternative evidence of identification to the satisfaction of the invigilators. Candidates failing to produce satisfactory evidence at the commencement of the examination will have their entry withdrawn.

After the examination the identification card must be retained for further use.

THE QUESTION PAPER
The paper will consist of 300 Multiple Choice Questions in book form. A computer Answer Sheet on which answers are to be recorded will be inserted into the Question Book and this sheet will be marked by a document reading machine. A sample computer Answer Sheet is shown overleaf. **You must use only the grade HB pencil provided for completing all parts of the Answer Sheets.** Pens must not be used for any part of the MCQ examination. Firm pressure is required with the pencil. You must ensure that your marking is bold and dark. You may erase any pencil mark by using the eraser provided. The time allowed for completion of the MCQ examination is TWO hours. You will be given a time warning 30 minutes and 10 minutes before the end of the examination. **Do not start the examination until instructed by the invigilator.**

FRONT COVER
On the front cover of each Question Book you must print your full name in the boxes provided and then sign your name in the space marked "signature". Your candidate number (not desk number) must be written in the FOUR SQUARES labelled "CANDIDATE NUMBER".

ANSWER SHEET (Sample overleaf)
A FIRM DARK IMPRESSION WHICH COMPLETELY FILLS EACH LOZENGE IS ESSENTIAL.

A FAINT LINE WILL NOT BE READ BY THE DOCUMENT READING MACHINE.

The Answer Sheet must not be folded, creased or torn. You must print your surname (family name) and other name(s) at the top of the Answer Sheet and write your CANDIDATE NUMBER in the boxes provided. Then **black-out** the lozenges corresponding to your candidate number.

YOU MUST SHOW YOUR NAME AS STATED ON YOUR ENTRY CARD.

ANSWERING THE QUESTIONS
The Answer Sheet is numbered 1-300 and against each number there are two lozenges labelled T(= True) and F(= False). You will be required to indicate whether you know a particular question to be true or false by **boldly** blacking out either the True or False lozenge.

To avoid too many erasures on the Answer Sheet, candidates may wish to mark their responses in the Question Book and then transfer their decisions to the Answer Sheet but this **must** be done **within** the two hours allowed for the examination.

Specimen questions and answers

When compared with radiotherapy, radical hysterectomy
1. is less favoured in stage 1a carcinoma of the cervix
2. carries a reduced risk of subsequent lymphocyst formation
3. allows preservation of ovarian function

Uterine curettage
4. is associated with an increased incidence of placenta praevia in a subsequent pregnancy
5. is important in the investigation of secondary infertility

Ovarian Thecomata
6. are typically benign

The following genital anomalies have a recognised association with the conditions listed:
7. Hypospadias : androgen insensitivity (testicular feminization syndrome)
8. Hypertrophy of the clitoris : maternal nortestosterone therapy
9. Varicocele : Klinefelter's Syndrome

In a patient with inappropriate lactation associated with secondary amenorrhoea
10. bitemporal hemianopia on perimetry would be expected in about 25% of patients
11. an exaggerated rise in serum prolactin concentration following injection of thyrotrophin releasing hormone is a recognised finding
12. an increased plasma concentration would be expected
13. treatment with Danazol would be appropriate
14. the administration of Methyl-Dopa is a recognised cause
15. anorexia nervosa is a recognised association

Answers 3, 6, 8, 11 and 14 are 'True'; answers 1, 2, 4, 5, 7, 9, 10, 12, 13 and 15 are "False". Your Answer Sheet relating to these questions would look like this when correctly filled in:

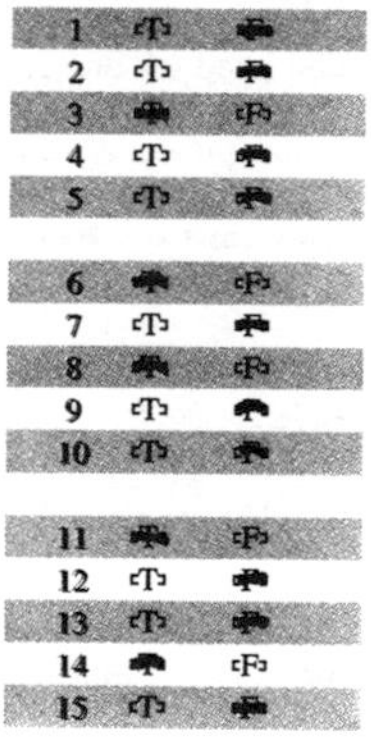

MARKING
Each question correctly answered (i.e. a True statement indicated as True or a False statement indicated as False) is awarded one mark (+1). For each incorrect answer no mark (0) is awarded. **All questions must be answered true or false. Incorrect answers are not penalised.**

COMPLETION
At the end of the examination, insert the completed Answer Sheet into the Question Book.

On no account may the Question Book be removed from the examination hall.

Any candidate who attempts to remove, by writing or by any other means, MCQ examination questions from the examination hall, will be reported to the Examination Committee and will FAIL the whole examination.

Royal College of Obstetricians and Gynaecologists
Part 2 Membership Examination

urname (Family Name) WILLIAMS

ther Name(s) PETER JOHN

Candidate Number

1	9	4	7
0	0	0	0
1	1	1	1
2	2	2	2
3	3	3	3
4	4	4	4
5	5	5	5
6	6	6	6
7	7	7	7
8	8	8	8
9	9	9	9

his form will be read by a machine
lease use the HB pencil provided
lark each answer with a single horizontal line T F
you make a mistake erase it completely
o NOT mark with ticks, crosses or circles
o not forget to enter your name and candidate number properly

T=True

F=False

IMPORTANT - When you have finished, check that you have answered EVERY question either true or false. If you leave any question blank it will be scored the same as an incorrect answer.

1	T	F	31	T	F	61	T	F	91	T	F	121	T	F
2	T	F	32	T	F	62	T	F	92	T	F	122	T	F
3	T	F	33	T	F	63	T	F	93	T	F	123	T	F
4	T	F	34	T	F	64	T	F	94	T	F	124	T	F
5	T	F	35	T	F	65	T	F	95	T	F	125	T	F
6	T	F	36	T	F	66	T	F	96	T	F	126	T	F
7	T	F	37	T	F	67	T	F	97	T	F	127	T	F
8	T	F	38	T	F	68	T	F	98	T	F	128	T	F
9	T	F	39	T	F	69	T	F	99	T	F	129	T	F
10	T	F	40	T	F	70	T	F	100	T	F	130	T	F
11	T	F	41	T	F	71	T	F	101	T	F	131	T	F
12	T	F	42	T	F	72	T	F	102	T	F	132	T	F
13	T	F	43	T	F	73	T	F	103	T	F	133	T	F
14	T	F	44	T	F	74	T	F	104	T	F	134	T	F
15	T	F	45	T	F	75	T	F	105	T	F	135	T	F
16	T	F	46	T	F	76	T	F	106	T	F	136	T	F
17	T	F	47	T	F	77	T	F	107	T	F	137	T	F
18	T	F	48	T	F	78	T	F	108	T	F	138	T	F
19	T	F	49	T	F	79	T	F	109	T	F	139	T	F
20	T	F	50	T	F	80	T	F	110	T	F	140	T	F
21	T	F	51	T	F	81	T	F	111	T	F	141	T	F
22	T	F	52	T	F	82	T	F	112	T	F	142	T	F
23	T	F	53	T	F	83	T	F	113	T	F	143	T	F
24	T	F	54	T	F	84	T	F	114	T	F	144	T	F
25	T	F	55	T	F	85	T	F	115	T	F	145	T	F
26	T	F	56	T	F	86	T	F	116	T	F	146	T	F
27	T	F	57	T	F	87	T	F	117	T	F	147	T	F
28	T	F	58	T	F	88	T	F	118	T	F	148	T	F
29	T	F	59	T	F	89	T	F	119	T	F	149	T	F
30	T	F	60	T	F	90	T	F	120	T	F	150	T	F

Check that you have answered every question either True or False.

This form will be read by a machine
Please use the HB pencil provided
Mark each answer with a single horizontal line [T] [F]
If you make a mistake erase it completely
Do NOT mark with ticks, crosses or circles
Do not forget to enter your name and candidate number properly

T=True

F=False

IMPORTANT - When you have finished, check that you have answered EVERY question either true or false. If you leave any question blank it will be scored the same as an incorrect answer.

151	[T]	[F]	181	[T]	[F]	211	[T]	[F]	241	[T]	[F]	271	[T]	[F]
152	[T]	[F]	182	[T]	[F]	212	[T]	[F]	242	[T]	[F]	272	[T]	[F]
153	[T]	[F]	183	[T]	[F]	213	[T]	[F]	243	[T]	[F]	273	[T]	[F]
154	[T]	[F]	184	[T]	[F]	214	[T]	[F]	244	[T]	[F]	274	[T]	[F]
155	[T]	[F]	185	[T]	[F]	215	[T]	[F]	245	[T]	[F]	275	[T]	[F]
156	[T]	[F]	186	[T]	[F]	216	[T]	[F]	246	[T]	[F]	276	[T]	[F]
157	[T]	[F]	187	[T]	[F]	217	[T]	[F]	247	[T]	[F]	277	[T]	[F]
158	[T]	[F]	188	[T]	[F]	218	[T]	[F]	248	[T]	[F]	278	[T]	[F]
159	[T]	[F]	189	[T]	[F]	219	[T]	[F]	249	[T]	[F]	279	[T]	[F]
160	[T]	[F]	190	[T]	[F]	220	[T]	[F]	250	[T]	[F]	280	[T]	[F]
161	[T]	[F]	191	[T]	[F]	221	[T]	[F]	251	[T]	[F]	281	[T]	[F]
162	[T]	[F]	192	[T]	[F]	222	[T]	[F]	252	[T]	[F]	282	[T]	[F]
163	[T]	[F]	193	[T]	[F]	223	[T]	[F]	253	[T]	[F]	283	[T]	[F]
164	[T]	[F]	194	[T]	[F]	224	[T]	[F]	254	[T]	[F]	284	[T]	[F]
165	[T]	[F]	195	[T]	[F]	225	[T]	[F]	255	[T]	[F]	285	[T]	[F]
166	[T]	[F]	196	[T]	[F]	226	[T]	[F]	256	[T]	[F]	286	[T]	[F]
167	[T]	[F]	197	[T]	[F]	227	[T]	[F]	257	[T]	[F]	287	[T]	[F]
168	[T]	[F]	198	[T]	[F]	228	[T]	[F]	258	[T]	[F]	288	[T]	[F]
169	[T]	[F]	199	[T]	[F]	229	[T]	[F]	259	[T]	[F]	289	[T]	[F]
170	[T]	[F]	200	[T]	[F]	230	[T]	[F]	260	[T]	[F]	290	[T]	[F]
171	[T]	[F]	201	[T]	[F]	231	[T]	[F]	261	[T]	[F]	291	[T]	[F]
172	[T]	[F]	202	[T]	[F]	232	[T]	[F]	262	[T]	[F]	292	[T]	[F]
173	[T]	[F]	203	[T]	[F]	233	[T]	[F]	263	[T]	[F]	293	[T]	[F]
174	[T]	[F]	204	[T]	[F]	234	[T]	[F]	264	[T]	[F]	294	[T]	[F]
175	[T]	[F]	205	[T]	[F]	235	[T]	[F]	265	[T]	[F]	295	[T]	[F]
176	[T]	[F]	206	[T]	[F]	236	[T]	[F]	266	[T]	[F]	296	[T]	[F]
177	[T]	[F]	207	[T]	[F]	237	[T]	[F]	267	[T]	[F]	297	[T]	[F]
178	[T]	[F]	208	[T]	[F]	238	[T]	[F]	268	[T]	[F]	298	[T]	[F]
179	[T]	[F]	209	[T]	[F]	239	[T]	[F]	269	[T]	[F]	299	[T]	[F]
180	[T]	[F]	210	[T]	[F]	240	[T]	[F]	270	[T]	[F]	300	[T]	[F]

Check that you have answered every question either True or False.

System Design by Speedwell Computing Services. 01604 410041

Mark Reflex® by NCSi NM-01317:654321 ED3803 Printed in

WARNING

BY OPENING THIS SEALED PACKAGE YOU ARE AGREEING TO BECOME BOUND BY THE TERMS OF THIS LICENCE AGREEMENT which contains restrictions and limitations of liability.

IF YOU DO NOT AGREE with the terms set out here DO NOT OPEN THE PACKAGE OR BREAK THE SEAL. RETURN THE UNOPENED PACKAGE AND DISKS TO WHERE YOU BOUGHT THEM AND THE PRICE PAID WILL BE REFUNDED TO YOU.

THE MATERIAL CONTAINED IN THIS PACKAGE AND ON THE DISKS IS PROTECTED BY COPYRIGHT LAWS. HAVING PAID THE PURCHASE PRICE AND IF YOU AGREE TO THE TERMS OF THIS LICENCE BY BREAKING THE SEALS ON THE DISKS, YOU ARE HEREBY LICENSED BY WB SAUNDERS COMPANY LIMITED TO USE THE MATERIAL UPON AND SUBJECT TO THE FOLLOWING TERMS:

1. The licence is a non-exclusive right to use the written instructions, manuals and the material recorded on the disk (all of which is called the "software" in this Agreement). This licence is granted personally to you for use on a single computer (that is, a single Central Processing Unit).

2. This licence shall continue in force for as long as you abide by its terms and conditions. Any breach of the terms and conditions by you automatically revokes the licence without any need for notification by the copyright owner or its authorised agents.

3. As a licensee of the software you do not own what has been written nor do you own the computer program stored on the disks and it is an express condition of this licence that no right in relation to the software other than the licence set out in this Agreement is given, transferred or assigned to you.

   Ownership of the material contained in any copy of the software made by you (with authorisation or without it) remains the property of the copyright owner and unauthorised copies may also be seized in accord with the provisions of the copyright laws.

4. Copying of the software is expressly forbidden under all circumstances except one. The one exception is that you are permitted to make ONE COPY ONLY of the software on the disks for security purposes and you are encouraged to do so. This copy is referred to as the back-up copy.

5. You may transfer the software which is on the disks between computers from time to time but you agree not to use it on more than one computer at any one time and you will not transmit the contents of the disks electronically to any other. You also agree that you will not, under any circumstances, modify, adapt, translate, reverse engineer, or decompile the software or attempt any of those things.

6. Neither the licence to use the Software nor any back-up copy may be transferred to any other person without the prior written consent of WB Saunders Company Limited which consent shall not be withheld provided that the recipient agrees to be bound by the terms of licence identical to this licence. Likewise, you may not transfer, assign, lend, rent, lease, sell or otherwise dispose of the software in any packaging or upon any carrying medium other than as supplied to you by WB Saunders Company Limited. The back-up copy may not be transferred and must be destroyed if you part with possession of the software. Failure to comply with this clause will constitute a breach of this licence and may also be an infringement of copyright law.

7. It is an express condition of the licence granted to you that you disclaim any and all rights to actions or claims against WB Saunders Company Limited and/or the copyright owner with regard to any loss, injury or damage (whether to person or property and whether consequential, economic or otherwise) where any such loss, injury or damage arises directly or indirectly as a consequence (whether in whole or part):

   a) of the failure of any software contained in these disks to be fit for the purpose it has been sold whether:
      i) as a result of a defect in the software, howsoever caused; or
      ii) any defect in the carrying medium howsoever caused; and/or

   b) any other act or omission of the copyright owner or its authorised agents whatsoever,

   and you agree to indemnify WB Saunders Company Limited and the copyright owner against any and all claims, actions, suits or proceedings brought by any third party in relation to any of the above matters.

8. This agreement is to be read as subject to all local laws which are expressed to prevail over any agreement between parties to the contrary, but only to the extent that any provision in this Agreement is inconsistent with local law and no further.

9. This agreement shall be governed by the laws of the United Kingdom.